"A welcome work of public opinion scholarship comparing what North Americans—on both sides of the Canadian/US border—think about their health care, their nation's programs, and what their neighbors have and do not have. This sharply contrasts with the mix of mischief and sheer mythology that prevails in much public debate."

—Ted Marmor, Yale University and Co-author of Politics, Health, and Health Care (2012)

"A fascinating, timely, and pioneering comparison of American and Canadian public opinion toward health policy. The authors use unique comparative survey data to explain how two broadly similar countries diverge in their views on health policy. Opponents of each country's system work overtime to frame flaws with a striking difference: most Canadians favor their system while many Americans welcome reform closer to the Canadian single payer model."

—Lawrence R. Jacobs, Mondale Chair for Political Studies, University of Minnesota

Health Care Policy and Opinion in the United States and Canada

Heated debate surrounds the topic of health care in both the United States and Canada. In each country, these debates are based in some measure on perceptions about health care in their neighboring country. The perceptions held by Canadians about the US health care system, or those held by Americans about Canada, end up having significant impact on health policy makers in both countries.

Health Care Policy and Opinion in the United States and Canada examines these perceptions and their effects using an extensive cross-national survey made up of two public opinion polls of over 3,500 respondents from the US and Canada. The book first develops a rigorous and detailed explanation of the factors that contribute to levels of satisfaction among Americans and Canadians with respect to their health care systems. It then attempts to study the perceptions of Canadians vis-à-vis the US health care system as well as the perception of Americans toward Canada's health care system. The authors examine how these perceptions impact health policy makers and show how the survey results indicate remarkable similarities in the opinions expressed by Americans and Canadians toward the problems in the health care system, heralding perhaps a measure of convergence in the future.

The authors present how perceptions on health care indicate elements of convergence or divergence between the views of Canadians and Americans and discuss how these citizen opinions should inform health care policy change in both countries in the near future. This book should generate interest in scholars of health care, public opinion, and comparative studies of social policies and public opinion.

Richard Nadeau is Professor of Political Science at the University of Montreal. His interests are voting behavior, public opinion, political communication, and quantitative methodology. A Fulbright Scholar, Professor Nadeau has authored or co-authored over 120 articles, chapters, and books including *French Presidential Elections* and *Le comportement électoral des Québécois* (Donald Smiley Award 2010).

Éric Bélanger is Associate Professor of Political Science at McGill University. His research interests include political parties, public opinion, and voting behavior. His work has been published in several scholarly journals including *Comparative Political Studies, Political Research Quarterly, Electoral Studies,* and the *European Journal of Political Research*. He is also the co-author of *French Presidential Elections* and *Le comportement électoral des Québécois*.

François Pétry is Professor and Chair of Political Science at Laval University. His main areas of interest are public policy, public opinion, comparative politics, and research methodology. He has published widely about the links between government policies and the preferences of citizens, as well as the use of polls in health care policy and election campaigning.

Stuart Soroka is Professor of Communication Studies and Faculty Associate at the Center for Political Studies, University of Michigan. His research focuses on political communication, the sources and/or structure of public preferences for policy, and the relationships between public policy, public opinion, and mass media. He is the author, among other work, of *Negativity in Democratic Politics* and *Agenda-Setting Dynamics in Canada*.

Antonia Maioni is Professor at McGill University in the Department of Political Science and the Institute for Health and Social Policy. From 2001 to 2011, she served as director of the McGill Institute for the Study of Canada, while also holding the position of William Dawson Scholar. She has published widely in the fields of comparative politics, public policy, and health care reform.

Routledge Studies in Governance and Public Policy

1 **Public Sector Ethics**
Finding and Implementing Values
Edited by Charles Sampford and Noel Preston with Carol-Anne Bois

2 **Ethics and Political Practice**
Perspectives on Legislative Ethics
Edited by Noel Preston and Charles Sampford with Carol-Anne Bois

3 **Why Does Policy Change?**
Lessons from British Transport Policy 1945–99
Jeremy Richardson and Geoffrey Dudley

4 **Social Relations and Social Exclusion**
Rethinking Political Economy
Peter Somerville

5 **Local Partnerships and Social Exclusion in the European Union**
New Forms of Local Social Governance?
Edited by Mike Geddes and John Benington

6 **Local Governance in England and France**
Alistair Cole and Peter John

7 **Politicization of the Civil Service in Comparative Perspective**
The Quest for Control
Edited by B. Guy Peters and Jon Pierre

8 **Urban Governance and Democracy**
Leadership and Community Involvement
Edited by Michael Haus, Hubert Heinelt and Murray Stewart

9 **Legitimacy and Urban Governance**
A Cross-National Comparative Study
Edited by Hubert Heinelt, David Sweeting and Panagiotis Getimis

10 **The Idea of Public Service**
Reflections on the Higher Civil Service in Britain
Barry O'Toole

11 **Changing Images of Civil Society**
From Protest to Government
Edited by Bruno Jobert and Beate Kohler-Koch

12 **Reasserting the Public in Public Services**
New Public Management Reforms
Edited by M. Ramesh, Eduardo Araral and Wu Xun

13 **Governing Modern Societies**
Towards Participatory Governance
Hubert Heinelt

14 Understanding the Politics of Pandemic Scares
An Introduction to Global Politosomatics
Mika Aaltola

15 Accountability in Crises and Public Trust in Governing Institutions
Lina Svedin

16 Democratic Governance and Social Entrepreneurship
Civic Participation and the Future of Democracy
Denise M. Horn

17 Health Care Policy and Opinion in the United States and Canada
Richard Nadeau, Éric Bélanger, François Pétry, Stuart Soroka, and Antonia Maioni

Health Care Policy and Opinion in the United States and Canada

Richard Nadeau, Éric Bélanger,
François Pétry, Stuart Soroka, and
Antonia Maioni

Routledge
Taylor & Francis Group
NEW YORK AND LONDON

First published 2015
by Routledge
711 Third Avenue, New York, NY 10017

and by Routledge
2 Park Square, Milton Park, Abingdon, Oxfordshire OX14 4RN

First issued in paperback 2016

Routledge is an imprint of the Taylor & Francis Group, an informa business

Library of Congress Cataloging-in-Publication Data

Nadeau, Richard, 1956–
Health care policy and opinion in the United States and Canada / by Richard Nadeau, Éric Bélanger, François Pétry, Stuart Soroka, Antonia Maioni.
pages cm. — (Routledge studies in governance and public policy ; 17)
Includes bibliographical references and index.
1. Medical policy—United States. 2. Medical policy—Canada. 3. Medical care—United States—Public opinion. 4. Medical care—Canada—Public opinion. 5. Public opinion—United States. 6. Public opinion—Canada. 7. United States—Foreign public opinion, Canadian. 8. Canada—Foreign public opinion, American. I. Bélanger, Éric. II. Pétry, François III. Soroka, Stuart Neil, 1970– IV. Maioni, Antonia. V. Title.
RA395.A3N2853 2015
362.1097—dc23
2014006301

ISBN 13: 978-1-138-21848-2 (pbk)
ISBN 13: 978-1-138-02108-2 (hbk)

Typeset in Sabon
by Apex CoVantage, LLC

Contents

Tables

Acknowledgements

This research project was a long time coming. The first discussions that some of us (Nadeau, Pétry, and Bélanger) have had about it took place nearly ten years ago, in 2005. The project took many turns in the years that followed, benefitting both from the addition of two collaborators (first Maioni, then Soroka) and the arrival of Barack Obama as US President. Our collective interests in comparative politics and in health care as a policy issue, as well as the health care reforms that are still under way south of our Canadian border, eventually coalesced into what we hope constitutes an interesting and stimulating comparative study of public opinion formation about health care in two neighboring countries.

This book would not exist, however, without the generous help of the Social Sciences and Humanities Research Council of Canada, in the form of a research grant awarded to Nadeau, Pétry, and Bélanger (grant number SSHRC 410–2007–0809). The development of our comparative survey questionnaire greatly benefitted from comments made on early drafts by Lisa Birch, Gerard Boychuk, Pierre-Gerlier Forest, Jennifer Jerit, and Ted Marmor. The help of three first-rate research assistants, Chris Chhim, El Hadj Touré, and Dominik Stecula, was crucial to the completion of the project. Finally, our editor at Routledge, Natalja Mortensen, has been a wonderful and unflinching supporter since our very first meeting with her. To all these people, our deepest and warmest thanks.

Introduction

Health care policies are an essential dimension of governmental action in advanced democracies. They are also an important concern for citizens—the issue has, after all, been at the heart of a good number of recent elections in both the US and Canada. Debates around eventual changes to any health care system will thus spark a great deal of interest from the public and the media. Under these circumstances, it is not surprising that political scientists have sought to better understand what moves public opinion on the issue of health care, and to what extent these opinion movements are likely to affect public policy in this sector.

A general interest in studying public opinion on health care has nevertheless resulted in what is thus far a relatively small body of work looking to understand the determinants of individuals' opinions on this issue. Our purpose in writing this book is to contribute to filling this gap in the literature by making use of a unique comparison, that of the US and Canada. Residing in neighboring countries with comparable economies and a common cultural and linguistic heritage, there are many similarities in Americans' and Canadians' political attitudes. Health care seems to be one exception. Although this was not always true in the past, today there are big differences in Americans' and Canadians' opinions toward their health care system. Americans are much less satisfied with their health care system than Canadians are with theirs. Americans are more likely than Canadians to demand significant health care reform. The demand for health care reform means something different to Americans and to Canadians. In Canada, where the health care system is publicly organized, demand for health care reform is stronger among those who prefer less government involvement in health care. In the US, where the health care system is privately organized, demand for reform is stronger among those who prefer more government involvement in health care. One final difference is that Americans feel a certain attraction toward the Canadian health care system whereas Canadians seem satisfied enough with their system and do not seem to be very attracted to the US system.

AMERICANS' AND CANADIANS' PERSPECTIVES OF THEIR HEALTH CARE SYSTEMS

The differences in Americans' and Canadians' opinions appear puzzling if one considers that the "objective" performance of the health care systems is rather similar in both countries. The personal experience of American and Canadian patients with their respective health care system is positive on the whole. Public perceptions of specific aspects of the health care system—precision of diagnosis and quick access to a specialist, surgery, or a hospital bed—are quite comparable in both countries; some of these perceptions are even more positive in the US today than in Canada (notably in wait times and in the possibility of quickly seeing a specialist).

To this day the divergence of opinion on health care in both countries has not received satisfactory explanation in the form of a single, all-encompassing empirical model. Explanations based on patients' personal experience with health care have been recently offered to account for the facts that Americans are less satisfied with their health care system and that they demand more significant health care reform than Canadians. One such explanation emphasizes discontent with the state of health care by large numbers of uninsured Americans (there are very few uninsured Canadians by comparison). Another explanation focuses more broadly on price rationing, the fact that the private, market-oriented American health care system limits the purchase of health care only to those buyers willing and able to pay the price (there is universal access to health care in Canada by comparison). A third explanation of the difference in public opinion about health care systems has focused on socioeconomic inequalities. Disparities in access to health care are more pronounced in the US than in Canada, and less-affluent individuals in the US are more likely to be deprived of health care and to express lower levels of satisfaction with the health care system.

Other researchers have linked higher levels of dissatisfaction with the health care system and stronger demand for reform in the US to political values and attitudes such as party identification or self-placement on a left–right ideological scale. Canadians who support the right-leaning Conservative Party are less satisfied with the status quo and are more likely to demand health care reform than those who support the left-leaning New Democratic Party. Inversely, Americans who support the Republican Party are more satisfied with the status quo and are less likely to demand health care reform than those who support the Democratic Party.

So far these explanations of the divergence of Americans' and Canadians' opinions toward their health care systems have only been offered in a scattered manner. What we have is an impressionist patchwork of results that are difficult to compare because they are based on different questioning, data, and methodologies. We have tried in this book to overcome these problems in two ways.

We have first articulated our analyses around three working hypotheses that encapsulate key questions about Americans' and Canadians' views on health care. First, we posit that individuals' basic needs and expectations in both countries about their health care system are, overall, quite similar. Second, we conjecture that Americans' and Canadians' opinions about health care are performance-responsive. Based on this notion, we expect (1) that socioeconomic variables will be more tightly linked to attitudes toward the health care system in the US than in Canada; (2) that affordability will be a greater concern in the US and wait times a more acute preoccupation in Canada; and (3) that the levels of satisfaction should be more performance-oriented in Canada (and more ideologically-oriented in the US) given that public health care provision is relatively similar across provinces. Third, and perhaps most importantly, we hypothesize that despite the fact that Americans and Canadians hold roughly similar views about the role of the state in general, the divergent orientations taken by the debates about health care in both countries—ideologically-oriented in the US and valence-oriented in Canada—go a long way toward explaining the marked differences between Americans' and Canadians' opinions regarding their health care system and that of their neighboring country. More specifically, we contend that the framing of the debates on health care, characterized by the central role of partisanship in the US and by varying commitments to equality in access to care in both countries, has left a significant imprint on Americans' and Canadians' views about the principles and the organization that should govern a fair and efficient health care system.

These working hypotheses tap dimensions that reflect both the demand side (individuals' needs and assessments) and supply side (partisan framing of the debate) of public opinion on health care. We expect that differences in opinions across borders will result from the interplay between these factors in the US and Canada. To put it more simply, we expect that despite similar needs and expectations about the performance of the health care system, Americans' and Canadians' views will differ and that this difference is mostly due to the way in which the debate about health care is framed in their respective country.

The second way in which we have tried to overcome problems in the existing literature is to provide more comprehensive and comparable results across the US and Canada. One drawback of the existing work is its lack of comparability and extensiveness. The results available are not only hard to compare but also are often incomplete, with too many missing interrelations between variables that potentially could be important. There has been little research effort at gathering together a large number of comparable explanatory variables in single multivariate models. This book aims to fill this research gap by building a multivariate model to explain the divergent perceptions by Americans and Canadians of their respective system of health. The data come from a detailed questionnaire administered online in the spring of 2011 to a little over 3,500 respondents in each of these two countries. To the best of our knowledge, this is the most complete and in-depth comparative study of public opinion conducted on this subject.

The opinion survey was administered at a time when there was a large difference in the intensity of the debate on health care reform. While the debate over health care reform was still in full force in the US in the spring of 2011 due to the recent adoption by the Obama administration of the Patient Protection and Affordable Care Act, discussions on health care reform, which had been at the top of the agenda a decade before, had lost much of their importance in Canada (though health care is still a top priority for a high proportion of Canadians according to many opinion polls). This asymmetry creates a situation allowing us to take into account the effect of the intensity of the debate—strong in the US, weak in Canada—on the determinants of opinion about the performance of the health care system and about what changes need to be put in place. To round out the comparison and ensure that the differences between the two countries are not solely due to the timing of the fieldwork, we will also take a brief look at the nature of the health care debate in Canada when it was at its height in the early 2000s.

One innovative aspect of this book is that it investigates in detail Americans' perceptions of the Canadian health care system as well as Canadians' perceptions of the American health care system. The interest in this comparison is twofold. First, it allows us the opportunity to see how citizens use certain decisional shortcuts to form their opinion regarding a health care system that they are only acquainted with in an indirect way. This opinion does not come from direct experience, but from an image of the health care system of the neighboring country perpetuated in one's own country and vice versa. Second, the comparison of Americans' and Canadians' opinions on the health care system of their respective neighboring country raises two important questions. First, what is the quality of public opinion in one country regarding a specific public policy of another country? Second, what is the impact of citizens' opinions of the health care system in the neighboring country on their attitudes toward health care reform in their own country? All other things being equal, is it possible that Americans having a positive image of the Canadian health care system could be more inclined to reform their own in a way that would bring it closer to the more universal Canadian one? The unique data from our comparative survey allows us to test this possibility, among others. Conversely, it is possible that Canadians having a positive image of the American health care system would be more inclined to reform their own in a way that would bring it closer to the more private nature of the American system.

The analysis will involve three distinct dependent variables, each one reflecting an aspect of public perceptions of health care systems: respondents' satisfaction with their own health care system, their impression of the health care system of the neighboring country, and their opinion regarding health care reform. For each of these three dependent variables, we will systematically test a model of opinion formation that includes successive "blocks" of explanatory variables: socioeconomic status variables, personal experience with the health care system and expectations about whether the system will be able to meet one's future needs, partisan preferences and opinions about state intervention, assessments of the health care system itself, and evaluations of the health system's past performance in general.

OVERVIEW OF THE BOOK

The book is divided into seven chapters. The first two chapters set the stage for our empirical study of health care opinion in the US and Canada. Chapter 1 offers a detailed explanation of the reasons why a comparison of Americans' and Canadians' views on their health care systems can be useful. It also presents our main theoretical approach based on the notion of issue framing, and distinguishes it from the other, more usual theories accounting for cross-border differences in public opinion in the US and Canada. The chapter then continues with a description of the public opinion data to be used in this book and the method used to analyze them. In particular, we explain in detail the logic of the multistage block-recursive approach that will be used to estimate the contribution of each group of factors to an explanation of Americans' and Canadians' satisfaction toward their own health care system, of their evaluation of their neighbor's health system, and of their propensity to support reform of their health care system.

Chapter 2 describes the national contexts in which opinions get formed. It starts by retracing the historical developments of health care policy in the US and Canada. It also draws a portrait of the current debates surrounding the health systems in the US and Canada. In doing so, it shows that the most recent debates in Canada were essentially about fixing the universally accepted, "iconic" public system (Boychuk 2008), whereas the battle on Obamacare involved intense and polarized views about the basic principles of the system itself (Jacobs and Callaghan 2013). Finally, the chapter describes the main characteristics of the health system delivery and financing in both countries. The contextual analysis offered in this chapter allows better understanding of the role of partisanship in health care attitudes and of the varying commitment to equality in access to care—two important factors that are shown to influence health care opinion in the next five chapters.

Chapter 3 begins by investigating, using mostly bivariate analyses, whether differences in personal attributes and experience with the health care system help explain cross-national differences in retrospective and prospective evaluations of both quality and access to health care services. We find striking similarities between the two countries—but some important differences as well. Canadians are concerned with wait times, whereas Americans are concerned with insurance. We find that the inability to afford health care clearly affects support of the health care system in the US. But the inability of the Canadian system to reduce wait times has negative effects on system support in Canada as well. The American and Canadian systems also share similarities: each is characterized by concerns about the future quality and availability of health care, although the distribution of these concerns is very different. In Canada moderate levels of concerns are shared equally across subgroups, whereas in the US inequalities in both concern about and access to health care are cumulative. One important message of Chapter 3 is that Americans' and Canadians' evaluations of their personal experiences with their health care system seem to largely overlap. These evaluations are nevertheless expressed in two different contexts: one where the constituent principles of the health care system are supported by a broad consensus (Canada) and the other where there is deep division about those principles (US).

Chapter 4 continues to use descriptive bivariate analyses to contrast the role that Canadians' consensual attitudes and Americans' polarized opinions play in their levels of satisfaction with the health care system. In Canada, we find that high levels of satisfaction with the health care system are correlated with a wide consensus around the broad principles underpinning the system. One way to interpret this correlation is that Canadians' relatively high levels of satisfaction are rooted in consensual values and attitudes about politics in general, and about health care policy in particular. Another way to look at it is that general satisfaction with the health care that the Canadian system delivers has contributed to developing further a consensus around those principles. By contrast, Americans' divided satisfaction with their health care system may be a reflection of their polarized political attitudes. Alternatively, the widely differential experience with the American health care system may have generated divided perceptions of satisfaction with that system. We also find that cross-border differences in attitudes are larger than within-country variations, a result that goes some way toward explaining cross-border differences in satisfaction levels. Finally, we argue that the perception of health care as a symbol of national unity has a unifying effect on satisfaction with the health care system in Canada. A similar unifying effect on satisfaction with the health care system fails to materialize in the US due to the absence of a perception of health care as a unifying symbol.

Chapter 5 presents a multivariate model of Americans' and Canadians' satisfaction with their health care system. The model brings together the socioeconomic, personal experience, ideological, partisan, and symbolic variables that were examined in a bivariate environment in the two preceding chapters. The results largely confirm those of Chapters 3 and 4. We find that satisfaction with the health care system is strongly affected by socioeconomic disparities in the US but less so in Canada. This finding is not unexpected given the large size and multifaceted impact of socioeconomic disparities in the US. We also find that satisfaction with the health care system is affected by regional disparities in Canada, but less so in the US. These last results, together with the bivariate ones presented in the previous chapter, offer new perspectives about the differences between Americans' and

Canadians' public opinion within and across borders. Among other things, the notion that North America might be meaningfully conceived as being formed of four sub-societies—English Canada, Quebec, US South, and US non-South (Grabb and Curtis 2005)—is disputed by our findings. Finally, assessments of the health care systems, based on both personal experience with them and an evaluation of their national performance, are also found to be important determinants of satisfaction with the health system in both countries, all else being equal.

Chapters 3, 4, and 5 focus on people's satisfaction with the health care system. This is appropriate in light of the central role that satisfaction plays in public opinion about health care system performance and about health care reform in the US and Canada. But another important question concerns cross-border perceptions of the health care system of their respective neighboring country. Recent debates surrounding health care reform in both the US and Canada have focused in part on the characteristics of the neighboring country's system. The Canadian system is seen as a model to emulate by many Americans who advocate change in their health care system, and vilified as "socialized medicine" by those who advocate the status quo. There is a similar reversed dynamics north of the border, where the private-market-oriented American system is glorified by some Canadians who advocate change, and demonized by most Canadians who want to keep the status quo.

Chapter 6 explores these ideas in further details by examining the determinants of Americans' and Canadians' perceptions of the health care system in the neighboring country. We find that Canadians largely have a negative opinion of the American health care system while Americans have a more positive view of the Canadian system. These opinions rest on well-entrenched perceptions about both systems. In the eyes of both Americans and Canadians, the main advantage of the Canadian health care system is its affordable care and universal coverage. In the eyes of many Americans, and some Canadians, the strengths of the American system are the possibility of quicker access to care and freedom of choice over one's doctor or hospital. We also find that citizens in each country have relatively clear opinions regarding health care policy in the other country. The evidence suggests that these opinions rest in part on factual knowledge. The comparison of factors explaining how Americans and Canadians evaluate their own health care system in addition to that of their neighboring country will allow us to assess questions with which citizens have direct experience and those with which citizens do not have direct experience.

Chapter 7 presents a multivariate model of Americans' and Canadians' support for health care reform in their country. At the outset, it should be emphasized that support for health care reform means something quite different to Americans and to Canadians. In Canada support for health care reform means support for an increase in the private sector's role in delivering health care and in providing health insurance. More generally, Canadians who support health care reform believe that there should be less government involvement in health care in Canada. In the US, support for health care reform at the time of our survey (spring 2011) meant support of a binding legislative framework that would ensure insurance coverage for all Americans. More generally, Americans who support health care reform believe that there should be more government involvement in health care in the US. In the end, we find that Americans are more likely than Canadians to demand significant health care reform. (This should come as no surprise knowing that Americans are generally less satisfied with their health care system than Canadians.)

Seymour Martin Lipset (1990, xiii) classically opined that the best way to learn about the US was to study Canada, and vice versa. We hope that the comparative analysis of public opinion in the US and Canada conducted in this book will go some way toward clarifying the factors behind the different opinion dynamics at play in these two neighboring countries.

1 Health Care Opinion across Two Countries

As was hinted at in the Introduction, and as our data will show in this chapter and in the remainder of this book, there is significant divergence between the US and Canada in the levels of public support for the health care system. Americans are less satisfied with their system despite similar assessments of the quality of medical care they personally receive. This general puzzle drives our empirical study of health care opinion in these two neighboring countries. It brings us to investigate a number of questions that our survey data analysis will aim at answering. First, what are the salient differences in the sources of public attitudes toward the health care system in these two countries, and in the determinants of public support for health care reform as well? Second, do Americans and Canadians hold different opinions about their neighbor's health care system, and do these opinions in turn affect the extent to which they would want their own system be reformed in one way or another? These are the core research questions that underpin this book.

COMPARING PUBLIC OPINION IN THE US AND CANADA

There have been a number of important in-depth studies that have compared health care policy in the US and Canada (e.g., Maioni 1998; Tuohy 1999; Boychuk 2008). These studies have been mainly concerned with identifying the various social, cultural, institutional, and political factors that can explain why the nature of the health care system in these two neighboring countries is so different. While we have learned much from them about the factors explaining these divergent policy outcomes—such as differences in political ideology or institutions, critical junctures and path dependence, and racial versus territorial integration policies—and although they have made a number of assumptions about differences between the two countries both in regard to public preferences concerning the optimal provision of health care as well as in regard to the role of public opinion in shaping public policy and vice versa, none of these studies have closely examined public opinion as well as its determinants.

Shall we expect convergence or divergence in American and Canadian public opinion about health care? It might be the case that the two publics display important similarities in their opinions about different facets of the health care system. In fact, it would not be the first time that such convergence in policy opinions would be observed between these two countries. Comparing public opinion in the US and Canada is particularly interesting because the two neighbor countries are very much alike with respect to the mix of issues in their respective public agendas. Likewise, Americans' and Canadians' public attitudes toward policy do share many similarities in a variety of policy domains (Mauser 1990; Mauser and Margolis 1992; Perlin 1997; Simpson 2000; Nesbitt-Larking 2002; Bélanger and Pétry 2005; Grabb and Curtis 2005).[1] There are powerful economic and social forces that appear to compel public opinion in the two countries toward similar sets of concerns and attitudes.

That said, as mentioned at the outset it seems more plausible to think that Americans and Canadians greatly differ in their attitudes toward their health systems. One reason may lie with the fact that the two countries present institutional differences that might lead us to expect differences in their opinion environment. For example, the Westminster-style parliamentary institutional system in Canada has remained very different from the American presidential system. The absence of checks and balances and the strong party discipline in the Canadian system have notably contributed to concentrate powers in the hands of the prime minister to an extraordinary degree (Savoie 1999). As a consequence, the Canadian government is able to control the public and the media agendas more often than the American government can (Soroka 2002; Bélanger and Pétry 2005), which may help foster greater support, or at least more deferential support, for the health care system in that country, as compared to what may be observed in the US with respect to public support for the health system.

Differences in institutions and, especially, cultures certainly go some way toward explaining the opinion divergence found between the US and Canada. Our own analysis will contribute in significant ways to strengthening this theoretical view, notably by introducing the idea that health care is a valence (and symbolic) issue in Canada whereas it is more of a positional (hence partisan) issue in the US. More generally, we propose that there are at least two important themes that influence public opinion in different, country-specific ways. The first involves the notion of equality. The US health system is highly unequal, particularly across income groups. Those with money have access, while those without money do not. The Canadian system is in contrast equal, but it provides equal access to "just better than mediocre" health care because the services need to be spread equally across all income groups, so to speak. The second crucial theme is partisanship. Health care in the US is a deeply partisan issue, with clearly defined camps, while in Canada it is not. Health care as an issue in Canada usually tends to cut across partisan groups, a phenomenon that acts as both cause and consequence of a relatively broad social consensus about the public nature of the Canadian health system.

In addition to these cultural aspects, which mainly refer to the demand-side dimension of public opinion about health care, we believe that an even more compelling account of health politics and public opinion in these two countries, and one that has been neglected so far in past studies, involves the extent to which the historic evolution of health policy and the broader political environment shape attitudes about health care policy in these countries. American and Canadian citizens compare their health system with that of their neighbor, and their political elites do the same in their efforts at building support for or against change in health policy. Hence, it is not possible to fully understand the dynamics of domestic health politics in each country without taking into account the impact of the neighbor's health care system, or at least the impact of public perceptions about it—perceptions that are, in part, the product of elites' issue-framing strategies.

This situation created by the geographic proximity of the US and Canada presents us with a rare (perhaps unique) case of citizens in one country having a relatively well-defined opinion regarding a specific public policy of another country. Obviously this opinion does not come from a direct experience with the neighboring country's health care system. Rather, it is the product of an image of the neighbor's health system that is perpetuated in one's own country and vice versa. As Marmor (1993) clearly showed, and as our own account of the evolution of American and Canadian health systems in the next chapter will reaffirm, debates on health care reform in the US have had reference to the Canadian health care system, seen as a model to imitate by those who advocate change and vilified as an example of "socialized medicine" by those who want to keep the status quo. The same dynamic also seems to be present on the other side of the border. For example, during the 2000 federal election, the incumbent Liberal government painted itself as a defender of the Canadian universal health care system and accused the main opposition party, the Canadian Alliance, of wanting to implement an "American-style" two-tier health care system in Canada against the wishes of an overwhelming majority of Canadians (Nadeau, Pétry, and Bélanger 2010).

Thus, opinions of Americans and Canadians regarding the health care system of their neighboring country are not artificial. They are in fact the product of the debates over health care reform in both countries where the characteristics of the neighboring country's system (or at the very least the characterization of it that is made) are invoked to justify either change or the status quo. The question that remains is whether these perceptions that citizens have of their neighbor's health system has any impact on their desire for health care reform. This is a question that has never been addressed directly by previous studies of American and Canadian public opinion—about health care or any other policy area. Our unique survey data will allow us to examine this issue and to assess whether citizens use these cross-country perceptions as decisional shortcuts to create an opinion about the necessity, or at least the desirability, to reform their own health care system.

As our analysis will show, Americans in favor of health care reform highlight the equitable nature of the Canadian system, and opponents highlight wait times and restricted choice. Similarly, proponents of change in Canada highlight the efficiency and flexibility of the US system, while the defenders of the Canadian system point out inequalities produced by the US system. This finding supports a large literature on the role of frames in the public opinion formation process (e.g., Chong and Druckman 2007; Delli Carpini and Keeter 1996; Schlesinger and Lau 2000; Zaller 1992). In other words, not only are the themes of equality and partisanship important to the way in which Americans and Canadians think about health care policy, but the framing of the health care debate by the political elites—around a cross-country comparison of the two health systems—actually accentuates the influence of these themes on public opinion, especially when it comes to attitudes toward reform. This process mainly constitutes the supply-side dimension of public opinion about health care, a dimension that we are particularly interested in bringing more to light in this book.

It is these broad notions about the usefulness of comparing American and Canadian health care systems, and the opinions that citizens hold about them, that anchor our empirical study of cross-national survey data. These notions will be further developed in Chapter 2 by looking at the historical evolution of the national contexts being studied. Then, Chapters 3 to 7 will propose more specific theoretical discussions and hypotheses, and will present our empirical results obtained with the methodological approach that we introduce in more detail in the upcoming two sections in this chapter.

We can note at the outset that our findings are noteworthy for several reasons. First, the findings contribute to our understanding of the determinants of public opinion in a policy area that occupies an important place in citizens' concerns. Second, debates surrounding health care in the US and Canada are based in some measure on perceptions about health care in the neighboring country. And these perceptions, whether or not they are based on actual fact, held by Americans about the Canadian health care system, or those held by Canadians about the US system, end up having a significant impact on health policy makers in both countries. Third, the results show some remarkable similarities in the opinions expressed by Americans and Canadians as to the problems in the health care system, heralding perhaps some measure of convergence in the future.

THE PUBLIC OPINION DATA USED

The book's empirical findings derive from an extensive cross-national survey, made up of two public opinion polls of a total of over 7,000 respondents from the US and Canada. More precisely, the opinion survey was simultaneously administered to 3,542 adult Americans and 3,522 adult Canadians by the polling firm Léger Marketing through Web-based interviews between February 3, 2011 and March 10, 2011. The survey's questionnaire was developed by the authors, and the fieldwork was financially supported by a research grant from the Social Sciences and Humanities Research Council of Canada.

The survey respondents were recruited in Canada via Léger Marketing's Légerweb online panel, and in the US via Western Wats' Opinion Outpost online panel. The median duration of the interviews was twenty minutes. A pre-test of 200 interviews (100 in each country) was performed in early January 2011 to validate the content of our questionnaire. Throughout the book, weighting procedures are used to ensure the representativeness of the samples in both countries. The weights are based on official data from the US Census and Statistics Canada about gender, age, region of residence, number of persons per household, and race (language in Canada).

The survey includes the most complete battery used to date to examine simultaneously the determinants of Americans' and Canadians' views about their health care system. It also contains a unique set of questions to assess the opinions of Americans and Canadians about the health care system of their neighboring country. A list of all the survey items used in our analyses is presented in the Appendix, together with information on how the answers were coded into variables.

Our empirical analyses will revolve around three main dependent variables: respondents' satisfaction toward their own health care system, their overall impression of the health care system in the neighboring country (the US for Canadians and vice versa), and their opinion regarding changes that should take place in their own health care system. The formulation of the questions for these three dependent variables is the following:

Satisfaction (Home): "In general, would you say you are very satisfied, fairly satisfied, neither satisfied nor dissatisfied, fairly dissatisfied, or very dissatisfied with the way health care runs in your country?"

Evaluation (Neighbor): "What is your overall impression of the health care system in Canada (the US): Very positive, moderately positive, moderately negative, very negative?"

Reforms (Home): "What approach would you say that this country's health system requires at present: a complete rebuilding from the ground up, some fairly major repairs, some minor tuning up, or is everything fine the way it is?"

The distributions of these three variables for the US and Canada are presented in Table 1.1. From this table, several findings can already be highlighted. First, the level of satisfaction toward the functioning of their own health care system is significantly higher in Canada than in the US. While 56% of Canadians state that they are very satisfied or somewhat satisfied with their system, this proportion is only 39% in the US.[2] This result may

Table 1.1 Opinions about Health Care in Canada and the US (%)

Panel A. Satisfaction		
	Canada	US
Very satisfied	12	8
Moderately satisfied	44	31
Neither satisfied nor dissatisfied	18	21
Moderately dissatisfied	18	24
Very dissatisfied	8	15
Don't know	0	1
Panel B. Neighbor		
	About US in Canada	**About Canada in US**
Very positive	2	17
Moderately positive	11	32
Moderately negative	38	12
Very negative	33	7
Don't know	15	32
Panel C. Reforms		
	Canada	US
Complete rebuilding	8	20
Major repairs	49	49
Minor tune up/everything's fine	39	26
Don't know	3	4

Notes: Sample sizes are 3,522 and 3,542 for Canada and the US, respectively. Data are weighted. After totaling the percentages, certain columns may not add to 100% because of rounding error.

partially reflect higher expectations on the part of American respondents in terms of what the health care system ought to deliver. If so, their satisfaction would be lower than Canadians' even if the systems in the two countries delivered identical results. A second finding is that Canadians collectively have a more assertive and negative opinion of the American health care system than the other way around, confirming the results of a recent Angus Reid study (Angus Reid 2009). In addition, we can observe that while 85% of Canadians actually express an opinion on the health care system of their neighbor country, this proportion drops to 68% in the US. Finally, Americans seem to want major change brought to their health care system, more so than Canadians. While 20% of Americans state that they want "a complete rebuilding" of their health care system, this percentage is only 8% in Canada. On the contrary, while close to two-fifths of Canadians state that they are satisfied with the status quo, barely one American in four (26%) has the same opinion.[3]

The information contained in Table 1.1 is reassuring because it falls in line with other studies on the collective opinions of Americans and Canadians regarding their health care system (notably, see Blendon and Taylor 1989; Blendon et al. 2002; Soroka, Maioni and Martin 2013). That said, while some of these results are known, the models that would allow us to systematically identify the determinants (socioeconomic profile, attitudes, motivations, perceptions) explaining the individual opinions underlying the distributions presented in Table 1.1 remain few and insufficiently developed. The rest of this book will be devoted to this task.

THE ANALYTICAL APPROACH ADOPTED

Our focus is on individual attitudes toward health care, and our aim is to modelize the factors that may influence these attitudes so as to gain a better understanding of the reasons why Americans and Canadians think the way they do with regard to issues of health care. Hence, our interest in this book lies in the cognitive process of opinion formation at the micro-sociological level. Whereas the presentation and analysis of aggregate-level data about the opinions of Americans and/or Canadians toward their health care systems are frequent both in the media and in academia, studies using micro-level data to analyze respondents' opinions on health care are relatively uncommon. In this context, the use of a "multistage block-recursive" model is helpful (Miller and Shanks 1996; Blais et al. 2002; Bélanger and Nadeau 2009; Nadeau et al. 2012).

A multistage block-recursive approach allows us to better establish the impact of a series of factors on these opinions, going from most distant on the causal path until they are the closest. This approach, which is reminiscent of the Michigan model used in the study of voting behavior (Campbell et al. 1960; Lewis-Beck et al. 2008), will focus here on five types—or blocks—of factors in the explanation of opinions on health care: (1) socioeconomic characteristics (age, gender, race, education, income, employment sector, region, Medicare recipient); (2) egotropic perceptions (past experience with the health care system and expectations about its future performance); (3) ideological and political preferences and attitudes (partisan identification, ideological position, individualism, preference of state intervention); (4) attitudes, opinions, and preferences dealing more specifically with health care systems (respective roles of the public and private sectors, symbolic value of the health care system); and (5) an overall assessment about the performance of the health care system in the past two years.

The five blocks' temporal sequence is easily justified. Socioeconomic status (SES) variables are the most distant factors since they capture individual characteristics that are temporally removed, for the most part, from personal experience with the health care system, from partisan preferences and opinions about state intervention, from attitudes about health care systems in general, from sociotropic assessments of the health care system itself, and from overall satisfaction with it. These socioeconomic variables are followed in the sequence by egotropic perceptions related to personal experience with the health system and expectations about the care to be received in the future (the second block of variables), by general ideological orientations and preferences (the third block), and then by more specific attitudes about health systems broadly speaking (the fourth block). The fifth and final block consists of an individual's assessment of the health system's past performance, which we label sociotropic perceptions.

As stated, the five blocks of explanatory factors are entered in the opinion model in successive steps (stages), from most distant to less distant. The general form of the multivariate models that will be used in the remainder of the book, and more directly in the last three chapters, will thus be the following:

> Opinion (health care) = *f* (SES, egotropic perceptions, general preferences, health care preferences, sociotropic perceptions).

The variables will be presented in the multivariate regression analyses according to the logic of block-recursive estimation. The first model will be estimated using only socioeconomic variables, and the other determinants (i.e., egotropic perceptions, general preferences, health care preferences, sociotropic perceptions) will then be successively introduced as blocks. Given the ordinal nature of our three main dependent variables of interest,[4] the most appropriate estimation method to use is that of ordered logistic regression (Wooldridge 2006). (Again, the specific codings of all our variables appear in the Appendix.)

This multistage block-recursive model of opinion toward health care will be directly tested in Chapter 5, which will explain satisfaction with one's own health system in each country. That multivariate analysis will build from the bivariate findings that will first be presented in detail in Chapters 3 and 4. Chapter 3 will examine the relationship between general assessments of the system on one hand and retrospective and prospective evaluations of both quality and access to services on the other. Chapter 4 will take a close look at the links between satisfaction with the system and views about its symbolic nature, as well as more general personal values and ideological preferences. These various explanatory factors will then be entered into a single model in Chapter 5 via multistage block-recursive analysis, controlling for the most distant factors (socioeconomic characteristics). The general multistage approach will be used again, with appropriate adjustments, in the final two chapters, which will deal with evaluation of the neighbor country's health system (Chapter 6) and with opinion about health care reform in one's own country (Chapter 7).

But first, Chapter 2 will describe in some detail the national contexts in which American and Canadian opinion about health care gets formed, allowing us to gain a better appreciation of the role of what we consider to be two key themes of the health care debate in both countries, equality and partisanship, as well as of the ways in which these themes have been framed by American and Canadian political elites in the past and in the current debates about health care reform.

NOTES

1. Though note that a contrary view emphasizing the differences in the policy attitudes of Americans and Canadians is offered by Lipset (1990) and Adams (2003). We further address this debate in Chapter 4.
2. The difference is statistically significant: chi = 316.88, p = 0.00.
3. The difference is statistically significant: chi = 293.85, p = 0.00.
4. Satisfaction with the health care system is a five-category variable (from very dissatisfied to very satisfied); opinion about the neighbor's health care system is a four-category variable (from very negative to very positive); and opinion about whether the country's health system is in need of reform is a three-category variable (from "everything is fine or just minor tuning up" to "complete rebuilding from the ground up").

2 The Evolution of Health Care Policy in the US and Canada

Before exploring the structure of public attitudes on health care in the US and Canada, we first need to understand the structure and history of the two health care systems. The aim of this second chapter is exactly that—a thorough account of the evolution of the two very different approaches to health care delivery.

The issues that citizens and governments in each country face today are heavily influenced by the past. This is true for a wide range of policy domains, of course—but even a brief review makes clear that it is particularly the case for health care. Accordingly, this chapter reviews the evolution of health care, first in the US and then in Canada, with a particular eye on two themes that are significant in analyses of public attitudes in subsequent chapters: the role of partisanship in health care attitudes and the varying commitment to equality in access to care.

THE EVOLUTION OF HEALTH CARE POLICY IN THE US

Despite the fact that Canada has had universal public insurance for several decades, forays into the debate over health insurance began earlier in the US. As early as 1910, the American Association for Labor Legislation led a campaign for health security that included cash payments and medical benefits for manual wage laborers (Numbers 1978). Introduced into several state legislatures, it received national attention after being endorsed by the Bull Moose Progressive Party during Theodore Roosevelt's campaign in 1912 (Walker 1969).

The Great Depression of the 1930s then traced the contours of a new cleavage in American partisan politics that would endure for decades to come. Although political parties and powerful interests were divided about the response to the economic crisis, public sentiment coalesced around the Democratic Party and Franklin Roosevelt's New Deal. The New Deal included a momentous milestone in American welfare state development, the Social Security Act. The Act included provisions for old-age pensions and unemployment insurance, but health insurance was conspicuously out of the picture—ostensibly a political choice based not so much on public opinion but on strategic opposition from stakeholders.

Compilations of public opinion on health insurance include some data for the 1936 to 1938 period, in which there is generally high support for government involvement in improving access to medical and hospital care (Schiltz 1970). For example, a 1938 Gallup poll found 81% of respondents supported government responsibility for providing medical care to those unable to afford it. There are other indications of a groundswell of support in the American public for economic reform and social insurance as well, including health care (Lipset 1983). And, indeed, the most voluminous amount of correspondence to the Congress had to do with prospects for health insurance, indicating support from a broad spectrum of the public, albeit with opposition coming mainly from physicians and American Medical Association (AMA)–affiliated state medical societies (Starr 1982).

Health insurance came back to the legislative agenda with Harry Truman in 1945 as part of his "Fair Deal" campaign. By then, opinion polls were showing over 50% of Americans in support of national health insurance initiatives (Schiltz 1970), despite considerable opposition from provider groups. Truman's plan, the first sent to Congress by a president, outlined a program in five points: hospital construction, public health, medical education and research, cash disability, and compulsory pre-paid medical care. Still, it proved to be a tough battle on Capitol Hill. The AMA was able to become a visible spokespiece for medicine and health interests, and became politically active in the 1946 midterm and 1948 presidential elections. Truman emerged from his narrow victory in 1948 even more determined to make health insurance his legacy to the nation, but the AMA response was directed not only at lobbying the Congress but also, more significantly, public opinion. A nationwide campaign was launched against "socialized medicine." To provide an effective alternative, the campaign suggested a renewed commitment to voluntary health insurance.

The $2 million campaign message linking compulsory health insurance with the dangers of communism was a decisive moment in turning public opinion around. Polls showed growing opposition to the Truman plan, with more support redirected at the AMA alternative. By the end of 1949, support for the administration plan had dropped to 36% (Schiltz 1970); by the 1952 election, it was dead as a legislative issue. This decisive defeat would have a profound impact on health insurance reform debate in the 1950s and beyond. In fact, at the same time that the federal government was backing away from legislative initiative, an expanding network of nonprofit, commercial, group, and union-sponsored health plans were emerging on the US market (Starr 1982). Thus, in the "wreckage" of the Truman proposals, reformers turned to a new approach that would target vulnerable groups shut out of the private insurance market.

For political reasons, the elderly emerged as the ideal target group. Social Security stakeholders were becoming an important political lobby in their own right, and public opinion at the time was generally in favor of aiding the elderly. The emergence of consensus around this limited approach to health insurance in the US would take a few years to solidify, but by the time the Democrats were back in power in 1960, the push to move forward had begun (Derthick 1979).

John F. Kennedy's victory was not considered a "mandate" for health reform per se, but health insurance would clearly be a primary feature of the administration's domestic agenda, setting in motion a public and legislative debate on health insurance. Polls showed steady support; a Gallup poll published in June 1961 indicated that 67% of Americans favored Medicare for the aged, even with increases in social security taxes, and the administration's private polling corroborated this widespread popularity (Jacobs 1992). Nevertheless, like Truman, Kennedy would be faced with a party divided on health insurance reform, a skeptical Congress, an openly hostile conservative coalition of Republicans and southern Democrats, and the powerful opposition of the medical lobby.

The medical lobby saw the measure as the precursor to government involvement in health care, alarmed by the British precedent (Derthick 1979) and the Canadian one as well (Maioni 1998). The AMA made extensive use of the "socialized medicine" threat in its public campaign against the measure. Still, legislators were nervous about such tactics: "it was one thing to write off socialism; but the risks of writing off the aged would give the wise politician second thoughts" (Marmor 1973, 28).

Indeed, partisanship had become key in the battle over health insurance for the aged. In 1964, President Johnson highlighted Medicare in his "Great Society" platform and voters responded overwhelmingly in favor: liberal Democrats won four seats in the Senate and forty-four in the House; in addition, almost all the doctors who ran for Congress lost (Sundquist 1968). Gallup polls following the election in December 1964 recorded 65% approval of Medicare. Public opinion had not changed dramatically since the first Kennedy initiative in 1961 (Schiltz 1970) but what had changed was how lawmakers perceived the political saliency of the issue.

What emerged was a "three-layer" compromise: in Medicare, the Democratic administration and reform proponents succeeded in compulsory hospital insurance for the aged; Republicans gained their proposals for supplementary medical insurance; and the AMA and insurers managed to get expanded government coverage of the medically indigent. This also allowed physicians to continue doing business as usual; initially, the only guideline being that they billed according to "reasonable charges."

Through Medicare and Medicaid, the US government took on the responsibility to guarantee access to health care for those groups most likely to be shut out of the voluntary and employer-based market for health insurance in the US. Liberal reformers had thought this would be the first step toward wider coverage and access, but the increase in the cost of health care and the explosion of public expenditures for health in the US led to a shift in the focus of health reform from improving access to health insurance to controlling the costs of health care. The Nixon administration's program for group-based health insurance was unsuccessful, although it did encourage the proliferation of Health Maintenance Organizations (HMOs) in the US.

Throughout the 1970s, Congressional Democrats, led by Senator Edward Kennedy, attempted to link access and cost concerns with renewed demands for national health insurance, but the enduring divisions within the Democratic Party on the issue, the hostility of the Republican opposition, and the persistent resistance of provider groups precluded such reform initiatives. Of note was the attempt to use the Canadian model as a way to promote national health insurance, even though the medical lobby in the US portrayed a "bitter" Canadian medical community, suffering from a "brain drain" of physicians south of the border.

The widespread reluctance to embark on new spending for entitlement programs and the neoconservative backlash pushed national health insurance out of the picture in the 1980s. Instead, reform was targeted at reducing federal expenditures, particularly Medicaid. Medicare was a more difficult target, since it enjoyed widespread public and political bipartisan support. The focus shifted to the regulation of the health services market by imposing changes and limits on payments to reimbursement. Private insurers, at the same time, began to impose greater restrictions on the type and extent of reimbursement they would cover.

In the run-up to the 1992 presidential race, health reform re-emerged, twinned to the fallout from a recession-wracked economy in which working Americans feared for their health benefits. Even the medical lobby, once a bulwark against government intervention, raised concerns about access to care, in particular the burden of caring for the uninsured and the limits imposed by insurers. Big business, saddled with a major portion of the American health bill, was increasingly frustrated by health cost increases and became another unlikely proponent of government regulation.

The Canadian model also played a part. A widely cited 1991 Government Accountability Office (GAO) report found that a single-payer system could save the US $3 billion of its health bill; others estimated this saving to be as high as $20 billion. Beyond the question of costs was the more fundamental question about the trade-off between quality and access. Detractors argued that Canada controlled health costs by limiting access to quality health care and freeloading off the US for research, innovation, and technology. And, of course, it was argued to be unfeasible by those who saw an incompatibility between Canada's political culture oriented toward government intervention and an American value system based on liberalism and individualism.

Whatever the merits of these competing arguments, widely debated in the public sphere, opinion polls showed a population very much in favor of some kind of reform. Bill Clinton's compromise, aimed at forging a middle path through the public regulation of private health insurance markets, explicitly rejected the single-payer alternative. The Health Security Plan of 1993 emphasized universal coverage through employer mandates and a mechanism for cost control through "managed competition" in health insurance markets; namely, government regulation of private insurers through regionally based "health alliances." The plan faced considerable opposition from powerful interests; insurance lobbies, in particular, waged effective campaigns that, like the medical lobby in previous decades, focused both on targeting legislators in both parties and influencing public opinion on a wider scale. Widespread public confusion ensued, heightened by the complex details of the President's health plan, the spectacle of warring factions on Capitol Hill, and the doomsday prophecies of its opponents. Even with a Democratic majority in the Senate, the bill was unable to move forward in 1994.

While far-reaching health reform was effectively swept off the legislative agenda, certain reforms moved forward that would have a significant impact on public health insurance programs. The Clinton administration's welfare reform package, for example, would lead to the development of SCHIP (State Children's Health Insurance Program) in 1997, a federal program that provided federal funds for the states to provide Medicaid coverage for children in low-income families. SCHIP quickly became the fastest-growing social program in the US, and within a decade over 5 million children were enrolled in it.

The 2000 decade was proving to be especially challenging on the health reform front. Overall health expenditures and per capita costs rose rapidly, as did employer-sponsored insurance premiums, at the same time that the US economy was shifting many workers into more precarious and part-time employment. The numbers of uninsured rose to over 45 million by 2005, one in six Americans (Bodenheimer and Grumbach 2012). Although the Republican administration in office did not pursue a health reform agenda per se—President George W. Bush would notably veto the expansion of SCHIP in 2007—the passage of the Medicare Modernization Act in 2003 was directed at trying to reduce the "gaps" in coverage that had become onerous for seniors. This included the option for recipients to choose a managed care plan under the Medicare Advantage program (Part C) and the creation of a Medicare Part D option to provide partial coverage of outpatient prescription drugs.

Despite these innovations, there was a considerable partisan divergence on the means and methods of health care reform, especially with regard to the conundrum between costs and access. This was also reflected in public opinion trends, which showed a firming of preferences more and more aligned with ideological precepts. Typically, a majority of Democrats were open to expanding coverage for the uninsured and undertaking more spending to effect substantive reform, while Republicans favored either more modest reform or the status quo.

These divisions became evident in the 2008 presidential race. Health care had become a dominant concern of middle-income Americans and a leading issue in the campaign. This was especially true among Democrats, who showed less satisfaction with their own care and more concern for the uninsured, even though health care was connected to a broader malaise about the American economy (Blendon, Altman, Deane, et al. 2008). Among the Democratic candidates, opinions diverged about the best way to open access to care. Senator Hillary Clinton, wearing the battle scars of the failed Clinton initiatives, turned from employer mandates to individual mandates that would require all Americans to be insured for health care. Her Republican rival, Mitt Romney, had introduced such a plan as governor of Massachusetts in 2006, requiring state residents to carry health insurance, aimed at reducing the burden of caring for the uninsured. Senator Barack Obama focused on children and families, making SCHIP expansion a focal point of his domestic policy platform, while his Republican opponent spoke more generally on the need for incremental change and cost control (Maioni 2009).

In public opinion analyses of both the primary season and the presidential face-off, the partisan divergences were striking (Blendon, Altman, Benson, et al. 2008). These were reinforced once it became evident that the new President, Barack Obama, intended to move as quickly as possible on health reform and was ready to expend the political capital to do so. And yet, as Obama's predecessors had learned, even the decisive majorities—53% of the presidential vote, Democratic control of both the House and the Senate—could not guarantee an easy run of it (Morone 2010).

By the time Obama addressed the Congress in September 2009, his message had firmed up considerably: "I am not the first President to take up this cause, but I am determined to be the last" (*New York Times* 2009). Obama's insistence on the basic elements of reform—insurance regulation, cost control measures, individual mandates—was crowded out by the deep divisions over the so-called public option. Here again, Canada entered the health care reform debate in the US, even though the single-payer model was no longer on any politician's agenda and the coverage of Canada was almost entirely negative. Parallels were made between the public option and the deficiencies of the Canadian system, while infamous ads featuring a Canadian "survivor" of the system and talk radio debates over "death panels" tried to illustrate the havoc that could be wreaked by constraining consumer choice and access. Although these attacks were as misleading as in the past, they resonated more powerfully because the debate over health care in Canada itself had changed, leading to a noticeable erosion of confidence among some Canadians.

To be sure, the eventual reform package was a "patchwork" in many respects, reflecting the complexities of the existing health system and the US political system itself (Marmor and Oberlander 2011). It is estimated that the new legislation would allow 32 million uninsured Americans to get coverage, with a price tag of over $900 billion (Bodenheimer and Grumbach 2012). Coverage would now be mandated, with health insurance exchanges and subsidies making it easier to find affordable insurance packages; regulation of insurers would be tightened; Medicare gaps would be addressed;

and access to Medicaid would be considerably expanded. But there would be no public option or opening toward "national" health insurance of the Canadian or European kind.

The passage of the Patient Protection and Affordable Care Act of 2010 (also referred to as ACA) was both a political coup and a hard-won compromise, reflecting not only active bipartisan cleavages (not a single Republican in Congress voted in favor) but also the nature of deeply divided public opinion on the matter, a situation that would persist into the 2012 electoral season. With a phased-in implementation timetable, through 2014, the Act provided ample room for subsequent challenges, including a Supreme Court reference in 2010. While the justices showed their own divisions on the matter, the major features of the Act held.

Still, we see here another interesting difference with Canada. The "national" character of the Canadian health care system is that, although each province and territory administers a health plan, everyone can expect to be covered for a comprehensive range of services, no matter where they live. The federal government is expected to chip in to make this happen and expects the provinces to play by its rule book in doing so. Intergovernmental friction has been a constant theme of fiscal federalism as a result, but the fracturing of the ACA is a different situation altogether. Indeed, the Supreme Court decision to curtail the federal government's obligation for states to expand their Medicaid coverage may lead to an even more "unequal" federal system in the US.

As can be seen from this brief overview of the historical development of health care policy in the US, the issue in that country tends to take on more of a "positional" character, especially in the last few decades. There is now deep division among the US public and elite about the constituent principles of the health care system (Jacobs and Skocpol 2012). This split tends to espouse the partisan cleavage found in that country, and even more so in recent years. Democratic politicians and supporters are more dissatisfied with their health care system and more in favor of reform, while Republican politicians and partisans appear more satisfied and are usually opposed to reforms, especially if their result were to bring the US health system closer to the Canadian one. Now that the Supreme Court has upheld the ACA, this partisan division will percolate at the state level in the years to come as critical yet often behind-the-scenes battles will rage over its implementation (Jacobs and Callaghan 2013). As the next section will make clear, in Canada partisanship has much less of a role in the health care debate nowadays than in the US.

THE EVOLUTION OF CANADIAN HEALTH CARE POLICY

Although medical associations in Canada were having similar discussions as in the US about European experiments in state medicine in the early 20th century, these did not translate into wider societal debates (Bothwell and

English 1981). By the 1920s, two things had changed: the federal Liberal Party endorsed social insurance after William Lyon Mackenzie King became leader in 1919 and, after the 1921 election, new protest parties in opposition upped the pressure for social reform, including Old Age Pensions that were passed in the midst of the constitutional crisis of 1926 (Bryden 1974).

Unlike the US, the onset of the Great Depression saw the absence of federal interest in health insurance, with Liberal Prime Minister King arguing about jurisdictional roles and financial capabilities, and his successor Conservative Prime Minister R. B. Bennett unable to do much beyond relief measures. Nonetheless, the impact of the Great Depression on public sentiment was significant, especially on lower- and middle-income families, both rural and urban, who were finding it increasingly difficult to pay for medical fees. Letters to Prime Minister Bennett illustrate starkly the toll the Depression was taking on people's health and ability to pay for care (Grayson and Bliss 1971). As the indigent medical care system collapsed, unpaid fees reached crisis proportions for the medical community as well, and members of the Canadian Medical Association were vocal in lobbying the federal government on the need for medical relief (Bothwell and English 1981).

Be that as it may, health care played little part in the Bennett "New Deal," the Employment and Social Insurance Act of 1935, which did little to prevent a Liberal sweep to office. Back in power, Prime Minister King chose not to implement the Act, instead referring it to judicial review that confirmed its infringement on provincial jurisdiction. A Royal Commission was announced to unravel these constitutional details, the fate of which would have a profound effect on encouraging a federal role in future social policy initiatives.

The weakness of Ottawa's responses to the Depression reinforced dissatisfaction with traditional parties in many parts of Canada, leading to the emergence of a new breed of protest parties, particularly in the west, and most significantly the Co-operative Commonwealth Federation (CCF), ready to articulate a social reform agenda in both federal and provincial politics. The presence of this new political element was to ensure that social reform agendas would continue to have a political voice.

The jurisdictional uncertainties that had plagued health and social initiatives in Canada during the Depression were addressed in the Royal Commission's 1940 report. The Commission agreed that health insurance was a provincial matter, but also maintained that there was a role for federal participation, at the request of the provinces, in both administration and tax arrangements, spurring considerable activity within the bureaucracy. A Committee on Health Insurance was tasked with soliciting the opinions of professional groups. In late 1942, it prepared a set of draft bills, including an enabling act authorizing federal contributions and a model bill for the provinces.

By this time, opinion polls had found that 75% of Canadians supported the idea of national health insurance (Canadian Institute of Public Opinion,

Gallup Poll, 8 April 1942). But the federal Cabinet remained divided, sensitive to the opposition of the medical profession and worried about the costs of such an initiative. At the same time, the CCF Party, making effective use of social reform issues, was rising rapidly in the polls, not only in the west but in Ontario as well. As such, the Liberal government was forced to pursue the commitment to a postwar social policy agenda. The fate of health reform was now in the hands of negotiations over a larger program of postwar economic and social reform that depended on federal-provincial agreement. When the intergovernmental talks over these measures broke down in 1945, so too did plans for health insurance.

The Liberal Party narrowly won the 1945 election, with its proposals for health insurance kept alive on its platform and in the House of Commons by the CCF. Aware of the potential of this third party in influencing public opinion and the need to do something on the health care front, the Liberal government enacted a National Health Grants program to be used for provincial efforts in infrastructure, research, and training.

Perhaps the most important development of that decade, however, was the election of a CCF government in the province of Saskatchewan and its subsequent passage of a hospital insurance plan in 1946. The emphasis on hospitals was suited to the rural character of the province. In addition, this form of government intervention did not directly interfere with the practice of private medicine, thus avoiding a direct confrontation with the medical lobby.

A few years later, public opinion polls started to show a substantial majority of Canadians in favor of government-financed hospital insurance: 62% of Canadians responded positively to an April 1956 Gallup poll that asked, "Would you favor, or oppose, a government-operated plan whereby any hospital expenses you incurred would be paid for out of taxes—even if it meant higher taxes?" By September, this margin had grown to 72%. In 1957, the federal government entered into the equation, this time at the request of many provinces, by setting up a cost-sharing program for hospital insurance.

By 1961, the ten provinces had introduced hospital insurance programs under the Hospital and Diagnostic Services Act and the stage was set for new innovations. The Conservative government in Ottawa had set up a Royal Commission to study health insurance in Canada but the CCF in Saskatchewan decided to go ahead with its own plan. The 1960 provincial election had turned into a referendum on that government's plan for medical insurance. Despite an intense public relations campaign on the part of Saskatchewan physicians, the CCF received a plurality of the vote and a majority of seats, which they took as a decisive mandate for action. A clash of wills was imminent, between the CCF on the one hand and organized medicine in Canada on the other. With a majority in the legislature, although the medical care insurance act was passed into law in 1961, its implementation was delayed due to a doctors' strike in the province in 1962. Most media in Canada and the US were highly critical of the doctors, more on the issues of ethics and legality than on the issue of medical insurance per se. The AMA, for its part, fighting its own battles against Medicare in the US, threw its support behind Saskatchewan doctors. Yet in the end it was the medical lobby that retreated first. Aware of rising public resentment throughout the province and the country, the strike ended three weeks after it began.

Meanwhile, in federal politics, the Liberal Party was taking a page out of the Kennedy handbook and redesigning its image into one of social reform. A new policy platform showcased medical care insurance, and the party kept close tabs on opinion polls, playing up health and social reform themes. By 1964, its margin of maneuver was narrowing, with the left-wing New Democratic Party (successor to the CCF) pushing for action in the House of Commons, and the Hall Commission report recommending a medical care plan along the lines of the Saskatchewan model. Concern about this Medicare initiative was not confined to the medical profession and its allies in business. There was also resistance in Parliament from more right-wing members and also from fiscal conservatives within the Liberal government. Nevertheless, as with Medicare in the US, medical insurance had become "politically potent; no one could afford to be seen as opposed" (Granatstein 1986, 196). And, indeed, the bill passed with multipartisan support in 1966, in stark contrast to the limited numbers of Republicans in the US Congress who voted for Medicare outright in 1965. Internal divisions with government, mainly over the cost implications of the new program, delayed its implementation until 1968. By 1972, all of the provinces had signed on to the shared-cost program. Quebec's proved to be the most distinct, based on integrating health and social services, and banning extra billing by physicians from the start.

The economic pressures of the 1970s forced the federal government to rethink the arrangement, shifting for open-ended cost sharing to block grants in 1977. This meant that cost control was now in the hands of the provinces. To ensure adherence to a form of national standards, the federal government passed the Canada Health Act in 1984, spelling out five principles for provincial health systems: universality, comprehensiveness, portability, public administration, and equal access. Despite the federal-provincial finagling and the transfer of power to a Conservative government in Ottawa that same year, politicians of all stripes supported the public insurance system. And with good reason, as health care was one of the most popular government-financed programs. The initial cross-national analyses by Blendon and his team (1989, 1990) showed the highest satisfaction rates among Canadians when compared to citizens in nine other advanced industrial countries.

Things began to change in the 1990s, as a stark economic climate and sharply reduced federal transfers put considerable financial pressure on the provinces, leading to rapidly implemented hospital closures, fee freezes or caps, and medical school reductions. The delivery of care quickly deteriorated, as exemplified mainly by longer wait times. Parallel to these changes, an erosion in public confidence was beginning to emerge (Maioni and Martin 2004). This growing dissatisfaction sparked a debate about the performance and the sustainability of the Canadian health care system, which reached its climax at the turn of the century (Mendelsohn 2002; Nadeau, Pétry, and Bélanger 2010).

The context of the early 2000s in Canada presents similarities with the debate over Obamacare ten years later. In both instances, health care was high on the public agenda, and significant proportions of the population were supportive of reforms. But the comparison ends there. A look at the state of public opinion in Canada in the early 2000s highlights the contrast between the two countries. In a 2002 report based on over 100 poll results, Mendelsohn emphasized that Canadians were very proud and attached to their health care system and that they were supportive of the Canadian Health Act and its core elements (for more public opinion evidence on this, see Chapter 4). He concluded his report by noting that Canadians, despite their growing perceptions in the 1990s about the deterioration of its performance, "like Medicare and think it should be preserved" (Mendelsohn 2002, vii).

A look at the reform agenda debated at the time is even more telling. To address the concerns of Canadians, the federal government established in April 2001 the Commission on the Future of Health Care in Canada to review Medicare. The Commission, headed by former Saskatchewan Premier Row Romanow, tabled its report in November 2002 after extensive consultations with health experts, provincial premiers and health ministers, health care workers, and the general public. The Commission pointed to a gap in health financing and services, in particular home care and national pharmacare, and the need to engage in major reform of primary care—but it also concluded from its work that strong leadership and improved governance is needed to keep Medicare a national asset (Romanow 2002).

The recommendations of the Romanow Commission are representative of the orientation of the debate about health care in Canada. Based on a detailed and careful review of the reform agenda in Canada for the period 1990–2003, Lazar (2009, 10) concluded that "a large majority of the reforms that were introduced, *or simply considered* were aimed at improving the existing health care model rather than replace it. In this sense, the love affair between Canadians and their health care system remained intact throughout the period covered" (our emphasis).

Even more revealing is the behavior of the political parties during that period. At the time of the 2000 federal election, health care was on top of the public agenda, and Canadians were dissatisfied with the performance of the governing Liberal Party on this issue (Mendelsohn 2002; Nadeau et al. 2010, 372–373). The literature about campaign strategies suggests that the incumbent government should have tried to redirect voters' attention away from health care so as to avoid the blame (Vavreck 2009). But the Liberals were actually able to campaign on that issue. Thanks to an ambiguous declaration made by the leader of the Canadian Alliance Party (their main opponent), the Liberals were able to portray the Alliance as being favorable to an "American-like" two-tier health care system. This strategy derailed the Alliance's campaign and made health care a winning issue for the Liberals (Nadeau et al. 2010; see also Blais et al. 2002). In a desperate attempt to counter the allegation that he was threatening the Medicare system, the Alliance's leader broke with the rules during the televised debate and held up a sign that read "No Two-Tier Health Care." This anecdote reveals better than anything else the political price to be paid when departing from the consensus about the Canadian health care system.

That lesson was well-taken by the successor of the Alliance, the Conservative Party, who since then has unquestionably backed the current Medicare system. Since coming to power in 2006, the Conservative government has, in fact, made it clear that health policy is a subject it wishes to avoid, being a matter of provincial jurisdiction in a worldview that sees social provision as a local, not national, matter. In this way, the Conservative government has dealt with recent health care issues through a stricter adherence to the formalities of fiscal federalism rather than the high politics of political partisanship over reform of the system.

To sum up, we note what appears to be a relative absence of a strict partisan story in the Canadian case in recent years, in contrast with the US. Partisanship, and especially the presence of a significant left-wing party in the form of the CCF/NDP, played an important role in Canada in the postwar period that saw the adoption of a universal health care system. But once that system was put into place, the political parties and most of the public rallied behind it.

DELIVERY AND FINANCING: CANADA AND THE US COMPARED

Through this historical development, every Canadian is now insured through a provincial government health plan, and every legal resident has access to publicly funded health care. These services are financed and regulated by the provinces, each with its own health legislation and administrative agencies, allowing for substantial autonomy at the sub-national level but, as the tensions in federalism suggest, a considerable fiscal burden as well. The federal government, meanwhile, takes on the costs of most refugee claimants as well as the health needs of aboriginal peoples, military and veterans, and inmates (although in most cases this care is devolved to the provinces), and also has a role in public health and safety.

All in all, however, only 70% of total health care spending flows through the public purse, mainly in the funding of "medically necessary" services that are delivered in a health care establishment and/or by a physician. First-dollar coverage ensures that co-payments, user fees, and extra billing cannot be imposed on publicly insured services. At the same time, many employers offer private supplementary insurance, but this is limited to services not covered by provincial plans (which can vary in this regard) such as optometry, dentistry, physiotherapy, some forms of diagnostic testing, and outpatient prescription drugs.

Canadian physicians, meanwhile, have conserved their autonomy insofar as they are mainly paid on a fee-for-service basis. Patients, too, tend to have a choice of physician, although in most cases they are required to have a referral from a primary care doctor before accessing specialist care. Physician fees, which vary across provinces, are negotiated between provincial medical associations and provincial public agencies. While fee-for-service medicine has been linked to medical inflation, billing in a single-payer system does have the advantage of reducing overhead. There are other notable advantages to this health system: Canadian physicians train at public universities at a relatively lower cost than their American counterparts, are covered by not-for-profit malpractice insurance, and operate in a legal system that constrains civil injury awards.

Of course, physicians must also abide by certain rules of the game and be prepared to work within the public system or opt out entirely. However, only a few specialized physicians in particularly lucrative domains do so, given the relatively low demand by private-pay patients and the need to access publicly funded hospitals to provide comprehensive care. In the past few decades, provinces have experimented with a number of measures to rein in physicians, including "caps" on billing, incentives to practice in less densely populated or more remote areas, and reductions in medical-school enrollment. Despite this, physicians' costs and their numbers are on the rise in Canada, even though imbalances in physician specialties and regional distribution persist. There are about 200 physicians per 100,000 Canadians today (around 70,000), comparable to the US but below the Organization for Economic Co-operation and Development (OECD) average (according to Canadian Institute for Health Information (CIHI) and Canadian Medical Association (CMA) data).

As in the US, hospitals in Canada developed over time as voluntary institutions (Boychuk 1998), often under religious or community auspices. Patients who are admitted to hospitals can expect all of their medically necessary services to be covered, including physician and nursing care, diagnostic procedures, drugs, anesthetics, and surgery and case room, as well as accommodation and meals (usually in a ward or semi-private room). Provinces may also offer other residential care (usually nursing home services) and home care as well.

Today, while hospitals remain independent, not government owned, they are expected to operate on a not-for-profit status. And, while a yearly global budget provides a stable and reliable funding source, not to mention significantly lower administrative costs, this also presents a considerable challenge for hospital administrators to live within a fixed income that may not account for spikes in demand. In addition, over the past two decades, while rates of hospitalization have decreased by almost a third, many hospitals have been forced to ration non-urgent care, particularly surgical interventions, in order to respect the principle of care based on priority of needs. With the new influx of funds garnered by the 2004 health accords, most provinces are now meeting wait-time benchmarks, although not entirely in the case of elective surgery, such as hip and knee replacement, for example (CIHI data).

Although the individual components of health care spending (e.g., share allocated to physician services, hospital care, prescription drugs) are comparable in Canada and the US, the dollar figures spent on health care are very different. Canada is a big spender among the OECD countries, with total spending on health care accounting for 11% of GDP (OECD 2011). After severe cuts in spending in Canada through the 1990s, growth in health care spending has been comparable to the US in recent years (about 4–5%).

In Canada, the pressure on the public purse is tied to overall fiscal pressure in the provinces, as well as the relative ability of government to fund other social programs. At the same time, however, it is the non-publicly funded areas, such as outpatient pharmaceuticals, that show rapid cost increases that put pressure on Canadian consumers. The American challenge is how to control the costs of a public system that exists within a competitive private market while attempting to make health care affordable overall and rein in total spending.

The US is still the most expensive health care system in the world, with 17% of GDP and almost $8,000 per capita, practically the double of what Canada spends. The key difference is that less than half these expenditures are accounted for by government financing. The majority of working Americans access health care through employer-sponsored insurance, for which they must contribute part of the premium. However, almost a third of Americans rely on government-financed programs. Those who have paid into Social Security are eligible for Medicare at age 65, although here too they contribute through deductibles and co-pays, and a premium for physician care and prescription drugs. The disabled are likewise able to access coverage through Medicare, even if under 65 years old. Those deemed medically indigent are eligible for Medicaid, jointly financed by the federal government and the states, while the children of poor families now have the option of enrolling in a SCHIP. While many of the previous criteria for Medicaid will be loosened with the new Affordable Care Act, it still remains a program for the lowest-income population.

Delivery of care itself is diverse and often dispersed. First, it must be noted that American states play a huge role in shaping health care—both public and private—in each state, with highly varying results and outcomes, such that the overall provision of health care in individual states probably varies more widely across states than it does among Canadian provinces. Second, most Americans are now enrolled in managed care plans, which are varied in scope and scale. This means that coverage can vary widely, and that physicians and hospitals earn income from a variety of different sources. The recent reforms will attempt to regulate insurance practice to some extent, but the connection between insurance and access remains the dominant model in the US health care system.

Will the Affordable Care Act narrow the gap between Canada and the US in the delivery and financing of health care? In a word, no. The same fault lines that we see reflected in public opinion over the years—and those that will be reflected in the analysis in this book—are likely to hold through the implementation of Obamacare. And this is because in Canada, despite the changes in funding and ongoing reforms in delivery of care, the essential components of a single-payer system across the provinces are still in place. The ACA, meanwhile, retains the multi-payer structure that has emerged in the US, in which Americans grapple with a wide variety of private options and public entitlements depending on their employment status, age, and income. The ACA arguably leads to even more complexity through the introduction of health care exchanges. In the end, too, concern about cost will likely retain significant differences between the two countries, mainly because the ACA does not, at least in the short term, address the fundamental challenge of cost control in a multi-payer system.

Indeed, the individual mandate further drives the differences with Canada by reinforcing the fundamental insurance principle—the care that you get depends on the type of coverage that you purchase—at the heart of access to care in the US. The ACA is designed to smooth out the most egregious inequalities in access and reduce the number of uninsured through insurance reform and subsidies to purchase affordable plans, but does not change the core conception about access to health services. Of course, it also means that Canadians will continue to grapple with the flipside of access based on need, namely waiting times for non-urgent care.

The new American law includes a review of Medicare reimbursement and the expansion of Accountable Care Organizations to reward cost-effective care. But it does not grapple in a systematic fashion with the overall inefficiencies in health care delivery and financing; the administrative burden of multiple payers, providers, and plans; and the cost pressures of defensive medicine. Governments in Canada know that health care is a searing financial responsibility, but they have at their disposal cost containment measures—monopoly fee negotiations with providers, global budgets for hospitals—that remain unfathomable in the American context.

Obamacare is a huge step in American health reform and, if seen to improve the system, will represent a major victory for Democrats. Like other major reforms of the past, however, it will entrench the private nature of the system and likely render national health insurance, or anything remotely like "Canadian-style" health care, impossible to attain.

CONCLUSION

The vast difference that exists between the US and Canada in terms of their respective approaches to delivery and financing of health care are rooted in different conceptions about equality of access, something that has become entrenched over the years through direct experience with the health care system. But that means that the health care system is constantly face to face with government decisions about financing, since delivery of health care depends on financing that involves redistribution of resources, so to speak, across the whole Canadian population, which may mean wait times in some instances. In the US, access derives from insurance coverage, which is conditioned by a number of different factors but, in the end, money plays a big role. Ultimately, both of these factors can impact health services.

This chapter has shown that there is similarity and difference in approaches to health care in the US and Canada. We have highlighted equality and partisanship as two of the most important themes that distinguish the American and Canadian cases, particularly in the current era. As will be seen in the remainder of this book, these themes have important incidence for our understanding of contemporary public opinion formation about health care in these two neighboring countries.

3 Satisfaction toward Health Care

Personal Attributes and Experience

Previous chapters have examined differences in the US and Canadian approaches to health care policy, as well as the general state of public attitudes about health care provision in both countries. This discussion has already spoken to the importance of history, and the structure of public policy, to public attitudes. That said, quite different systems can lead to (some) relatively similar results. This is the theme of the current chapter.

The chapter begins by reviewing some general assessments of the system in both the United States and Canada. It compares results across countries, and distinguishes between retrospective and prospective evaluations of both quality and access to services. Results highlight some of the differences between the two, but some striking similarities as well. In short, in both countries, there are serious concerns about access to health care; that said, those concerns are a product of quite different access-to-services issues, and that means that the exact nature of access concerns in Canada is different than in the US. In Canada the concern is wait times, while in the US it is insurance.

We explore attitudes on both issues here, and connect access-to-services concerns—and experiences—with general assessments of system quality. As we shall see, an inability to afford health care clearly matters to system evaluations and support. In this regard, the American system presents some serious difficulties. But the Canadian system suffers from long wait times—and waiting for access quite clearly has deleterious effects on system support as well. Indeed, insofar as a public system is dependent on public support, the inability of the Canadian system to reduce wait times may be particularly problematic.

For all their differences, then, the US and Canadian systems also share some similar traits. Each is characterized by moderate levels of support, by concerns about future quality and availability of care, and by the negative impacts of wait times and/or a lack of insurance. One of the more striking differences between the two systems is in the distribution of these concerns, however. In Canada, moderate levels of concern are shared equally across subgroups, while the US shows more marked inequalities in both concern about and access to health care. *This* is, we believe, a central difference between the systems. It will, we hope, become clear in the sections that follow.

GENERAL ASSESSMENTS: THE QUALITY OF CARE

Table 3.1 provides a starting point for a comparison of personal experiences with health care in the US and Canada. The table shows results from the general question, "Overall, how do you rate the quality of medical care that you and your family have received in the past 2 years from your doctor/GP/the place you usually go to?" Results are striking. First, overall, the quality of health care in both countries receives relatively good grades. Only 6.3% of Canadians and 4.4% of Americans select the responses "poor" or "very poor." Second, differences in assessments across the two countries are very minor. Indeed, when responses are coded into a 0–1 scale, the average score in the US and Canada is the same (0.69).

The similarity in overall assessments of the quality of care is interesting given the many differences between the two countries' health care systems. How can health care models be so different, but outcomes—at least where satisfaction is concerned—be so similar? There is more than one way to skin a cat, of course; it may well be that two quite different systems produce outcomes that in the end are relatively similar. But it may also be that lying behind these relatively similar assessments (and many other similar assessments in forthcoming tables), there are some significant differences.

Indeed, results in the chapter that follows suggest that this is the case. Retrospective assessments of services may be relatively similar in the US and Canada, but the weaknesses in health care provision and the sources of concern amongst citizens are actually quite different. In short, high overall levels of satisfaction with the quality of care in the US obscure large differences amongst those with and without insurance. This, according to survey responses at least, is the critical weakness in the US system. But the Canadian system is not without its weaknesses as well. As we shall see, universal access has come at the cost of longer wait times in Canada.

Table 3.1 Quality of Services

	Canada	US
Mean Satisfaction (0–1 scale)	0.69	0.69
Excellent	19	17
Very good	47	49
Fair	28	29
Poor	4	3
Very poor	2	1

Notes: Sample sizes are 3,522 and 3,542 for Canada and the US, respectively. Cells contain percentages based on weighted survey data. Question Wording: Overall, how do you rate the quality of medical care that you and your family have received in the past 2 years from your doctor/GP/the place you usually go to?

RETROSPECTIVE AND PROSPECTIVE ASSESSMENTS OF SERVICES

We begin our examination of differences in assessments across the US and Canada by looking at results from three questions capturing respondents' retrospective assessments of services. The full question wording for each of three retrospective questions is included in the top panel of Table 3.2, alongside the results.

Table 3.2 makes clear again that the gap between the US and Canadian systems is not especially large. Roughly one-quarter of respondents in each country recall "a time when you felt that you or a member of your family needed health care buy you didn't receive it." The percentage is slightly higher in Canada than in the US in this case.[1] Responses to the other retrospective questions point in the opposite direction. Roughly one-quarter of US respondents recall "a time you or a member of your family were unable to receive the most effective drugs you needed," as opposed to 14% in Canada.[2] And there is a small, three-point gap between the percentage of Americans and Canadians who recall "a time you or a member of your family were unable to receive high quality medical care."[3]

Table 3.2 Retrospective Assessment of Services

	Canada	US
General Assessments		
During the past 2 years . . .		
. . . was there ever a time when you felt that you or a member of your family needed health care but you didn't receive it? (% yes)	27	23
. . . was there ever a time you or a member of your family were unable to receive the most effective drugs you needed? (% yes)	14	24
. . . was there ever a time you or a member of your family were unable to receive high quality medical care? (% yes)	19	22
Access to and Use of Services		
At the moment, do you have a family doctor? (% yes)	85	73
Have you or a member of your family needed non-emergency or elective surgery in the past 2 years? (% yes)	29	27
How many times have you or a member of your family used a hospital emergency department in the past 2 years?	2	1

Notes: Sample sizes are 3,522 and 3,542 for Canada and the US, respectively. Cells contain percentages based on weighted survey data.

These relatively small differences in retrospective evaluations are reflected in questions on system use as well, in the bottom panel of Table 3.2. There is a significant difference in the percentage of respondents who say they have a family doctor—85% in Canada, and 73% in the US.[4] But system use suggests somewhat smaller gaps. Twenty-nine percent of Canadians say yes to "Have you or a member of your family needed non-emergency or elective surgery in the past 2 years?"; the corresponding percentage in the US is 27%.[5] The average response to "How many times have you or a member of your family used a hospital emergency department in the past 2 years?" in Canada is 1.9; in the US, 1.3.[6]

In short, while cross-country differences in retrospective evaluations are statistically significant, they are rather small in magnitude. Two of the general assessments questions reveal three-point differences pointing in opposite directions. The questions on "the most effective drugs" and on having a family doctor are the only ones pointing to what we regard as substantively different responses. In each case, results clearly favor the Canadian system. (Though note that the difference for drugs cannot be a function of the Canadian health care system, which does not include pharmaceutical coverage. It may have to do with supplementary plans offered by employers, or other factors, we cannot easily tell.) This fits with what we see in prospective evaluations as well. Indeed, when thinking about future care, differences across the two countries are more striking. Those differences also all point in the same direction. Again, full question wording is included alongside results in the table. The first two questions are prospective versions of two access questions framed retrospectively in Table 3.2—access to the "most effective drugs" and ability to "receive high quality medical care." Response categories are different for these prospective questions—there are four responses: very high, fairly high, fairly low, and very low. Table 3.3 shows the proportion of respondents selecting either very high or fairly high in response to the questions asking about the risk of a lack of access in the future. In both cases, roughly one-half of Americans express concern about future availability of services, whereas in Canada the percentage concerned is 34% and 39%, respectively.[7] A second set of questions asking about respondents' confidence in the health care system in the event that they are seriously ill captures a similar cross-national gap. In each case, a greater percentage of Canadians are "very confident" or "somewhat confident" that they will have access to services. The gap is relatively small (roughly five percentage points) for the three questions focusing on access. The final question, asking about whether respondents will "be able to afford the care you need" reveals a wider, fifteen-point gap in confidence.[8] And a final question capturing "worry" about future health care coverage finds a twenty-point gap.[9]

Overall, results from prospective questions in Table 3.3 point to a difference across the US and Canada that was not clearly in evidence in the general assessment of care reviewed in Table 3.1. Retrospective assessments of the two health care systems are relatively similar, but Americans clearly

Table 3.3 Prospective Assessment of Services

	Canada	US
General Assessments		
In the coming years . . .		
. . . do you think that the risks that you or a member of your family may be unable at one time or another to receive the most effective drugs you needed are (% very high + % fairly high)?	34	49
. . . do you think that the risks that you or a member of your family may be unable to receive high quality medical care are (% very high + % fairly high)?	39	48
How confident are you that if you become seriously ill, you will . . .? (% very confident + % somewhat confident)		
. . . get quality and safe medical care	81	76
. . . receive the most effective drugs	80	72
. . . receive the best medical technology	75	71
. . . be able to afford the care you need	70	54
When you think about the coverage of your health care needs and those of your family in the future, would you say that you are (% not worried at all + % not very worried)?	53	33

Notes: Sample sizes are 3,522 and 3,542 for Canada and the US, respectively. Cells contain percentages based on weighted survey data.

worry more about future access to care than do Canadians. The difference may not be surprising given the current debate about the health care system in the US. But Canadians, too, are in the midst of a debate about the future viability of health care, and commentators have regularly highlighted what appear to be major flaws in the long-term viability of the system. The comparisons in Table 3.3 have put Canadians' ongoing concerns about the future quality and availability of health care in context.

ISSUES OF ACCESS: WAIT TIMES

This is not to say that Canadians' concerns are not justified. The system is quite clearly under pressure, and nowhere has that pressure been more apparent than in the debate about wait times. And there are significant differences in wait times across the US and Canada. Table 3.4 shows results from questions tapping general assessments of wait times, as well as questions asking about recalled wait times for both elective surgery and emergency room visits. The general assessments make the difference between the US and Canada

Table 3.4 Wait Times

	Canada	US
General Assessments		
Over the past 2 years, have you or a member of your family had to wait longer than you thought was reasonable to get health care services? (% yes)	50	31
In the coming years, do you think that the risks that you or a member of your family will have to wait longer than reasonable to get health care services are . . . (% very high + % fairly high)	67	54
Recalled Waiting Times		
Surgery: After it was decided that a surgery was needed, how many days, weeks or months did you or a member of your family have to wait for the non-emergency or elective surgery?	10th perc: 4 Mean: 117 90th perc: 270	10th perc: 3 Mean: 52 90th perc: 60
Emergency rooms: The last time that you or a member of your family went to an hospital emergency department, how long did you wait before being treated?	10th perc: 1.0 Mean: 4.4 90th perc: 9.0	10th perc: 1.0 Mean: 3.0 90th perc: 5.0

Notes: Sample sizes are 3,522 and 3,542 for Canada and the US, respectively. Cells contain row percentages, based on weighted survey data.

readily apparent. There is a nearly twenty-point difference in the percentage of Canadians versus Americans who recall waiting longer than "was reasonable" to get health care services.[10] Indeed, roughly one-half of Canadian respondents recall such a wait. And two-thirds of Canadians (14% more than in the US) believe that the likelihood of unreasonable wait times in the future is either very or fairly high.[11]

These general assessments mirror recalled wait times. The table shows the average recalled wait time for those scheduled for elective surgery and for emergency room visits; the 10th and 90th percentiles are also shown. The gap in elective surgery wait times is striking: the mean wait time in Canada (117 days) is more than twice as long as in the US (52 days), and the 90th percentile in Canada is roughly 9 months long. Emergency room wait times show a similar trend: the mean in Canada (4.4 hours) is more than a third longer than in the US (3.0), with a 90th percentile of 9 hours. Clearly, Canadians both recall and experience much longer wait times than do Americans.

Where issues of access are concerned, this appears to be the major issue in the Canadian case. Wait times are markedly longer than they are in the US, at least for emergency room access and elective surgery. This may well not be the case for acute care services, of course—those experiencing a heart attack in Canada, for instance, seem to receive quick and effective care (Soroka and

Fournier 2011). This is as we should expect when resources are limited—however, triage means that more critical cases can receive good care at the cost of less critical cases. But the system-wide impact of lower levels of service for less critical cases may be decreasing public faith in and support for universal care (see, for example, Soroka 2007).

Decreasing public support as a function of wait times has been shown elsewhere (Soroka and Fournier 2011), but it is especially clear in our data, shown in Table 3.5. The table shows responses to questions capturing both retrospective and prospective assessments of the health care systems. These are the same questions reported in Tables 3.2 and 3.3—but here, mean responses are reported for those saying they did or did not wait longer than they thought was reasonable for services. In every case, those who waited longer for services offer lower evaluations of the system. The impact of waiting is slightly greater in Canada than in the US. This may have to do with the salience of wait times in the current Canadian health care debate, but it may also be related to the fact that wait times in Canada are simply much longer than in the US—waiting longer than was "reasonable" quite clearly means more in Canada. But the fact that wait times also matter in the US makes clear that Canadians are not unique in their reaction to lack of ready access to services.

Perhaps more importantly, while the impact of waiting is weaker on prospective assessments than on retrospective assessments, it is substantively

Table 3.5 The Effects of Waiting on Retrospective and Prospective Assessments

	Canada		US	
	Retrospective Assessment	Prospective Assessment	Retrospective Assessment	Prospective Assessment
Did not wait	2.89	2.50	2.84	2.18
Waited	2.43	2.20	2.52	1.94
Difference	*–0.47*	*–0.30*	*–0.32*	*–0.24*
Significance (t)	*–16.66****	*–14.05****	*–10.82****	*–10.05****
N	3,404	3,422	3,430	3,417

Notes: Sample sizes are 3,522 and 3,542 for Canada and the US, respectively.

***$p < 0.001$; **$p < 0.01$; *$p < 0.05$.

Waiting: Over the past 2 years, have you or a member of your family had to wait longer than you thought was reasonable to get health care services?

Retrospective Assessment (1–5): In your opinion, has access to health care in your country over the past two years . . . greatly deteriorated (1), deteriorated (2), stayed the same (3), improved (4), or greatly improved (5)?

Prospective Assessment (1–4): What approach would you say that this country's health care system requires at present . . . complete rebuilding (1), fairly major repairs (2), minor tuning up (3), everything's fine (4)?

large and statistically significant in both countries. It makes good sense that a poor experience with the system would decrease retrospective assessments. But it also affects respondents' expectations for the future. Decreasing expectations and support, as a function of wait times, may be a central concern for the current Canadian system.

ISSUES OF ACCESS: INSURANCE

Where the Canada–US comparison is concerned, we should not lose sight of the fact that lower wait times in the US are reported by those who have access to health care. There is no simple way to compare wait times that include indefinite waits by the insured, but including those quite clearly present a different picture of the relative advantages of one system over the other. In short, both systems suffer from problems of access. In the Canadian case, access issues revolve around wait times; in the US, they are focused on insurance.

Table 3.6 shows responses to questions on health insurance. The Canadian question is relatively simple—it is not about whether they have access to health insurance, but rather whether they have private insurance in addition to the existing universal plan. Roughly 70% of respondents do; the remaining 30% rely only on the government-funded system.

The situation is rather more complex in the US. There are five questions capturing different ways in which Americans may be insured—through their

Table 3.6 System Access: Coverage

Types of Coverage		
Canada	Any private health insurance such as insurance that is paid by you, your family, your employer, an association or some combination thereof (% yes)	69
US	Health insurance through your or someone else's employer or union (% yes)	51
	Medicare, a government plan that pays health care bills for people aged 65 or older and for some disabled people (% yes)	24
	Medicaid or other state medical assistance plan for those with lower incomes (% yes)	15
	Health insurance you bought directly (% yes)	16
	Health insurance from another source (% yes)	15
No Coverage		
US	Current (based on questions above)	16
	Recent: In the past year, was there ever a time when you did not have any health insurance coverage? (% yes)	24

Notes: Sample sizes are 3,522 and 3,542 for Canada and the US, respectively. Cells contain percentages based on weighted survey data.

employer or union, Medicare, Medicaid, insurance paid for by themselves, or another source. Note that these categories are overlapping—a given individual may have various forms of insurance from multiple sources. We cannot simply add up the percentage in each category to find out how many Americans have insurance (indeed, the percentages add up to over 100%). The bottom panel of Table 3.6 thus shows calculations for the number of uninsured individuals. Roughly 16% of respondents give negative responses to all five insurance questions—these individuals are entirely uninsured. Taking into account the possibility that respondents can be intermittently uninsured (because they lose their job, for instance) points to larger problems. Nearly one in four Americans were uninsured at some point in the year 2010.

US respondents' reported satisfaction with various insurance plans does not seem to vary widely. Table 3.7 shows results from a question asking

Table 3.7 Satisfaction with Insurance (US only)

	Mean Satisfaction (0–1 scale)	Very Satisfied	Fairly Satisfied	Fairly Dissatisfied	Very Dissatisfied
All respondents	*0.60*	18	54	15	12
Respondents by insurance plan*					
Health insurance through your or someone else's employer or union	*0.64*	18	61	15	6
Medicare, a government plan that pays health care bills for people aged 65 or older and for some disabled people	*0.66*	23	56	16	5
Medicaid or other state medical assistance plan for those with lower incomes	*0.54*	13	51	21	15
Health insurance you bought directly	*0.60*	12	62	19	7
Health insurance from another source	*0.65*	18	63	16	3

Notes: Sample sizes are 3,522 and 3,542 for Canada and the US, respectively. Cells contain percentages based on weighted survey data, based on the question, "Overall, are you very satisfied, fairly satisfied, fairly dissatisfied or very dissatisfied with your current insurance plan?" Percentages for each type of insurance plan in the US are based on respondents with that plan type only (i.e., excluding respondents with more than one type of insurance plan).

Table 3.8 Difficulties with Insurance

	% Yes	
	Canada	*US*
. . . obtaining payment exemptions or the right to special rates for health care	14	14
. . . completing or filling out applications for health insurance	11	11
. . . finding out what benefits you are entitled to from your own health insurance plan	17	22
. . . getting reimbursement from a health insurance organization	15	15

Notes: Sample sizes are 3,522 and 3,542 for Canada and the US, respectively. Cells contain percentages based on weighted survey data, based on the question, "In your dealing with private health care organizations, have you had any difficulties . . .?"

about satisfaction with insurance plans. The mean score is 0.60; Medicaid appears to receive the lowest level of satisfaction; Medicare the highest. Note that the scale for this question is different and thus not directly comparable, but it is worth noting that overall levels of satisfaction with insurance plans in the US are not fundamentally different from overall levels of satisfaction with the health care system in both the US and Canada, shown in Table 3.1.

Indeed, Table 3.8 points to relatively small differences between the US and Canada where difficulties with insurance are concerned. Insurance in the US does appear to present more problems than insurance in Canada, but only marginally more so. In fact, none of the differences in Table 3.8 are statistically significant.[12] To the extent that Americans suffer at the hands of insurance companies, Canadians do as well. In each case, roughly one in five respondents expressed a concern with finding out what benefits they were entitled to, for instance. There is a critical difference, however: in the Canadian case, insurance covers services in addition to the public system—no Canadian has to figure out if their insurance covers critical surgeries, for instance. In the US, the same is not true. Difficulties in determining benefits may occur at relatively similar levels from one system to the next then, but the consequences in the US are clearly much greater.

This is more readily apparent in Table 3.9, which shows results from questions on payment for services. Almost all questions show a roughly twenty-point gap between the US and Canada. Americans are much more likely to report having paid for services, of course. They are also much more likely to have not received care due to a lack of money and to be concerned about receiving care in the future for similar reasons.[13]

What is the impact of a lack of insurance on system support? Table 3.10 examines the relationship between insurance and system support. It does so by repeating the analysis already seen in Table 3.5, for wait times. Here, we look at mean assessments, both retrospective and prospective, based on those with or without insurance.

Table 3.9 Payment for Services

	Canada	US
Have you or a member of your family ever paid a non-refundable out-of-pocket payment for a medically necessary service such as a consultation with a doctor, a hospital service, a procedure or diagnostic test at a private clinic? (% yes)	38	49
Would you say that this payment was (% very high)	16	29
During the past 2 years, was there ever a time you or a member of your family did not receive the care needed because you were unable to afford it? (% yes)	11	27
In the past 2 years, did you or a member of your family have any problems paying medical bills or not? (% yes)	9	34
In the coming years, do you think that the risks that you or a member of your family might not be able at one time or another to afford needed health care are (% very high + % fairly high)?	36	58
When you think about paying for the costs of your medical care and those of your family in the future, including your insurance premiums, would you say that you are (% worried + % somewhat worried)?	49	70
All things considered, are you very satisfied, fairly satisfied, fairly dissatisfied or very dissatisfied with the total costs you're paying personally to get your medical care and that of your family? (% very satisfied + % fairly satisfied)	77	57

Notes: Sample sizes are 3,522 and 3,542 for Canada and the US, respectively. Cells contain percentages based on weighted survey data.

The impact of insurance is not exactly directly comparable across the two systems—we are after all talking about supplementary insurance in the Canadian case. Even so, the impacts of insurance on system support are in some regards relatively similar. In each case, the impact of insurance on retrospective evaluations is not so clear. In the US, there is no significant impact; in Canada, those with insurance show marginally lower retrospective evaluations. (It may be that poor views of the system are part of what drives Canadians to opt into additional insurance.) The impact of insurance on prospective assessments is clear in both systems, however: in both cases, prospective assessments of the health care are markedly lower for those without insurance. This is not at all surprising in the US case—clearly, those who must pay out of pocket for health care (except perhaps for the very wealthy, an issue we explore further) will be less supportive of the existing system. We regard the impact of a lack of insurance in the Canadian case as particularly interesting, however. Here, we are talking about additional insurance that covers the costs of drugs, dental care, and other services such

Table 3.10 The Effects of Insurance Coverage on Retrospective and Prospective Assessments

	Canada		US	
	Retrospective Assessment	Prospective Assessment	Retrospective Assessment	Prospective Assessment
Without insurance	2.75	2.47	2.37	1.94
With insurance	2.62	2.79	2.34	2.13
Difference	*–0.13*	*0.32*	*–0.04*	*0.19*
Significance (t)	*–2.09**	*–8.19****	*–0.03*	*–7.10****
N	3,404	3,422	3,430	3,417

Notes: Sample sizes are 3,522 and 3,542 for Canada and the US, respectively.

***p < 0.001; **p < 0.01; *p < 0.05.

Retrospective Assessment (1–5): In your opinion, has access to health care in your country over the past two years . . . greatly deteriorated (1), deteriorated (2), stayed the same (3), improved (4), or greatly improved (5)?

Prospective Assessment (1–4): What approach would you say that this country's health care system requires at present . . . complete rebuilding (1), fairly major repairs (2), minor tuning up (3), everything's fine (4)?

as physiotherapy or massage therapy. These gaps in the public system clearly have an impact on public support.

In both countries, then, insurance matters to system support. Just as in the US, those without insurance in Canada are more likely to believe that the system needs rebuilding. That said, the fact that insurance increases support in both countries should not distract us from an equally if not more important fact: overall assessments of the health care systems, particularly prospective ones, are markedly lower in the US than in Canada. Table 3.10 is relatively clear in this regard: a lack of insurance moves the mean prospective assessment in Canada from roughly 2.8 to 2.5; it moves the same assessment in the US from 2.1 to 1.9. Regardless of insurance, Americans see a greater need for health care reform than do their Canadian counterparts.

INEQUALITY IN ACCESS TO HEALTH CARE

What accounts for Americans' greater support for reform, even as they express roughly similar assessments of their quality of care? First, note that most of the preceding results are based on national averages and do not distinguish between those who do and do not have ready access to care. Table 3.11 makes clear the importance of distinguishing between the two

Table 3.11 Views of the Uninsured

		Canada	US
Overall, how do you rate the quality of medical care that you and your family have received in the past 2 years from your doctor/GP/the place you usually go to? (mean satisfaction scale, 0–1, as in Table 3.1)	*All respondents*	0.69	0.69
	Respondents with insurance only	0.70	0.71
	Respondents with no insurance only	0.66	0.57
During the past 2 years, was there ever a time you or a member of your family did not receive the care needed because you were unable to afford it? (% yes)	*All respondents*	11	27
	Respondents with insurance only	9	23
	Respondents with no insurance only	15	51

Notes: Sample sizes are 3,522 and 3,542 for Canada and the US, respectively. Cells contain means or percentages based on weighted survey data.

groups. The table shows results for two of the questions used—one on overall assessments of the quality of care, the other on a lack of access to care due to an inability to pay for it. In each case, we distinguish between (1) all respondents, (2) respondents with insurance only, and (3) respondents without insurance only.

The impact of insurance on the quality and availability of care in each country is readily evident. Assessments of the quality of care are lowest amongst those with no insurance. In Canada, however, the difference is slight; in the US, there is a twelve-point drop. The frequency with which respondents report an inability to afford care shows a similar trend. In each case, the percentage of those saying yes to the question doubles as we move from those with insurance to those without—but the shift in Canada is 9% to 15%, and in the US it is 23% to 51%. Clearly, the 15–20% of Americans without insurance are receiving markedly less care.

The gap is wider still when we take income into account. A lack of insurance is less problematic for those with high incomes, of course. An overwhelming majority of respondents without insurance are in the lowest income bracket, obviously. Even so, just 11% of those who lack insurance and are in the highest income tercile in Canada say "yes" to the question about not being able to afford care—much more similar to the insured than the uninsured group in Table 3.11. But 17% of those who lack insurance and are in the lowest income tercile in Canada say "yes." In the US, 54% of those who lack insurance and are in the lowest income tercile say "yes."[14]

Table 3.12 makes much more explicit the differences in both satisfaction with and access to care across demographic subgroups. The table shows results for the same variables used in the preceding table, but here we see means broken down by gender, age, education, income, employment, and race.

Table 3.12 Satisfaction and Lack of Access to Care, by Demographics

	Satisfaction with Care		Lack of Access to Care	
	Canada	*US*	*Canada*	*US*
Gender				
Female	0.69	0.69	12	33
Male	0.69	0.70	9	22
Age				
18–34	0.65	0.66	14	32
35–54	0.67	0.68	12	30
55+	0.75	0.75	7	18
Education				
HS or less	0.68	0.68	13	32
More than HS	0.69	0.69	11	29
Completed university	0.71	0.72	8	20
Income				
Lowest tercile	0.68	0.65	16	37
Middle tercile	0.70	0.71	10	26
Highest tercile	0.71	0.74	5	16
Employment				
Government employee	0.72	0.73	11	24
Non-government employee	0.66	0.70	10	25
Self-employed	0.71	0.69	14	35
Employer	0.63	0.68	13	27
Not working (incl. student, homemaker)	0.73	0.70	10	28
Race				
White	0.70	0.71	10	26
Other	0.63	0.65	13	31

Notes: Sample sizes are 3,522 and 3,542 for Canada and the US, respectively. Cells contain means or percentages based on weighted survey data. Question Wording: *Satisfaction:* Overall, how do you rate the quality of medical care that you and your family have received in the past 2 years from your doctor/GP/the place you usually go to? *Lack of Access to Care:* During the past 2 years, was there ever a time you or a member of your family did not receive the care needed because you were unable to afford it? (% yes).

Differences in satisfaction with medical care over the last two years are relatively small from one subgroup to the next. As we have already seen, overall levels of satisfaction are similar in the US and Canada. There is a greater degree of variance in the US case, however—the mean value is in this case produced by a combination of low levels of satisfaction from those without access to care combined with somewhat higher levels of support from those with ready access. We can start to see the difference that income makes here, however: the shift from the first to third income tercile matters in both countries, but somewhat more in the US.

Differences across both subgroups and countries are more readily apparent in the question asking about whether respondents did not receive care because they were unable to afford it. Overall levels are higher in the US, as we have already seen. But differences across subgroups are more striking as well. There is a ten-point gender gap, where women are more likely to report lacking care; younger respondents are twice as likely to report a lack of care than are older respondents; there is a twelve-point gap across education cohorts and employment groups; and a five-point gap across racial groups (we collapse non-whites here due to sample size).

Many of these differences are almost certainly related to the impact of income. Even in Canada, moving from the lowest to highest income tercile leads to a ten-point drop in reported lack of care. But the gap in the US is twice that size. Sixteen percent of those in the highest income tercile report not having received care due to cost, compared to 37% of those in the lowest tercile. This is the core difference between the two health care systems. Each produces similar overall levels of support, but support in the US is highly contingent on a combination of insurance and income.

CONCLUSION

Broad similarities in satisfaction with the provision of health care in the US and Canada clearly mask some important differences between the two systems. Both systems grapple with issues of access, but the nature of the problem is quite different: in Canada, the concern is wait times; in the US, it is access to insurance. And inequalities, across income groups in particular, are much more apparent in the US case. We will be addressing these inequalities again in the next chapters. For the moment, we turn to an exploration of some other important determinants of public satisfaction toward health care, namely, political values and attitudes.

NOTES

1. The difference is statistically significant: chi = 12.03, p = 0.00.
2. The difference is statistically significant: chi = 123.46, p = 0.00.
3. The difference is statistically significant: chi = 10.54, p = 0.00.
4. The difference is statistically significant: chi = 64.34, p = 0.00.
5. The difference is statistically significant: chi = 4.15, p = 0.04.
6. The difference is statistically significant, based on a two-tailed t-test of means: t = 7.1340, p = 0.00.

7. Based on all four categories, both differences are statistically significant: chi = 249.42, p = 0.00; chi = 116.38, p = 0.00.
8. Based on all four categories, all differences are statistically significant: chi = 64.69, p = 0.00; chi = 122.93, p = 0.00; chi = 73.89, p = 0.00; chi = 373.44, p = 0.00.
9. Based on all four categories, the difference is statistically significant: chi = 510.96, p = 0.00.
10. The difference is statistically significant: chi = 287.10, p = 0.00.
11. The difference is statistically significant: chi = 190.65, p = 0.00.
12. Tests of significance are, in the order in which questions are presented in Table 3.8: chi = 0.004, p = 0.95; chi = 0.46, p = 0.50; chi = 3.28, p = 0.07; chi = 1.68, p = 0.20.
13. All cross-country comparisons are statistically significant. They are, in the order in which they are presented in Table 3.9: chi = 89.67, p = 0.00; chi = 77.32, p = 0.00; chi = 324.73, p = 0.00; chi = 711.81, p = 0.00; chi = 505.67, p = 0.00; chi = 551.19, p = 0.00; chi = 389.66, p = 0.00.
14. These results are not shown in detail here.

4 Satisfaction toward Health Care

Values and Symbols

This chapter investigates how Americans' and Canadians' political values and attitudes correlate with their satisfaction with the health care system. It argues that higher satisfaction in Canada versus the United States cannot be primarily explained by marked differences in fundamental political values and attitudes. True, Canadians appear somewhat more favorable to government intervention than Americans are, but (as we shall see) these differences are not particularly important and could not account for the large satisfaction gap toward the health care system observed across both countries. Even as Canadians and Americans tend to converge on basic political principles, however, they hold rather divergent views about the basic principles on which their health care system should be based. Canadians express strong support for a single-payer universal health care system (Medicare in the Canadian sense), whereas Americans appear more divided about the merits of their market-based system.

This chapter will document this puzzle by showing that Americans' and Canadians' attitudes are quite similar on basic political principles, but at odds about health care. We will also show that both types of political attitudes, either general or issue-specific, can be tightly linked to the level of satisfaction toward the health care system in the US. We will finally argue that stronger correlations in the US reflect the intense partisan polarization over health care and explain in turn the lower level of satisfaction observed in this country.

The results presented in this chapter are consistent with our expectations outlined here. We have suggested that health care is a valence issue in Canada and a positional one in the US. If this line of reasoning is correct, we should find stronger correlations between political attitudes and opinions on health care in the US. The different status of the health care system in both countries, "iconic" in Canada and "partisan" in the US, explains why Americans' and Canadians' levels of satisfaction toward their health care system differs so much. Canadians tend to view their health care system as a symbol of national unity; American citizens clearly do not. The status of the Canadian health care system as national symbol generates loyalty from the part of many Canadian citizens. This loyalty is translated into support of, and satisfaction with, their health care system, irrespective of their level of satisfaction with the health care they receive.

The next section of the chapter examines correlations between general political values and attitudes in the US and Canada such as party identification, left-right (or liberal-conservative) ideology, individualism, perception of what the role of government ought to be in society, and the level of satisfaction toward the health care system in each country. It is argued that these variables have an important polarizing effect on Americans' satisfaction with their health care system, but that they only have a very weak effect on Canadians' satisfaction with their health care system. Put differently, health care in the US is a highly partisan issue; in Canada, it is not.

Subsequent sections explore how satisfaction is correlated with political values and attitudes that are directly related to health care. It is argued that Canadians' consensual political attitudes about health insurance and access to health care have a strengthening effect on their satisfaction toward their health care system, whereas Americans' polarized attitudes on these topics have a weakening effect on Americans' satisfaction with the health care system. We will then examine the correlation between satisfaction with the health care system and Canadians' and Americans' perceptions of health care as a unifying symbol. Both Canada and the US are very large countries with strong regional variations in policy attitudes in general and attitudes toward health care in particular. Therefore, we ask in the last section of this chapter whether some of the variables we associate with satisfaction with health care are influenced by these regional variations.

GENERAL POLITICAL VALUES AND ATTITUDES

Recall that our survey data make clear that Canadians are significantly more satisfied with their health care system than Americans (Table 4.1). As already seen in Chapter 1 (Table 1.1), according to our survey, 56% of Canadians who have an opinion on this issue are "very" or "fairly satisfied" with their health care system, 18% are "neither satisfied nor dissatisfied," and 26% are "very" or "fairly" dissatisfied. By comparison, only 39% of Americans are satisfied, 21% are neither satisfied nor dissatisfied, and 39% are dissatisfied with their health care system. Moreover, attitudes are polarized in the US, with equally large numbers of Americans satisfied and dissatisfied (39% in both cases) with their health care system. In Canada, a clear majority is satisfied; indeed, twice as many Canadians are satisfied (56%) than are dissatisfied (26%) with their health care system.[1]

This section examines the distribution of some ideological/political attitudes in the US and Canada and pays particular attention to the relationship between these variables and Americans' and Canadians' satisfaction with the health care system. Two findings stand out from these analyses. First, it appears that citizens of both countries share many things in common when it comes

Table 4.1 Quality of Services and Satisfaction with the Health Care System

	Canada			US		
	Very/Fairly Dissatisfied	Neither Satisfied nor Dissatisfied	Fairly/ Very Satisfied	Very/Fairly Dissatisfied	Neither Satisfied nor Dissatisfied	Very/ Fairly Satisfied
Very/ fairly poor	70	14	16	75	19	6
Fair	37	27	36	54	26	20
Very good/ excellent	16	15	69	31	19	50

Notes: Sample sizes are 3,522 and 3,542 for Canada and the US, respectively. Data are weighted. $\chi 2 = 229.5$ with 2 df; $p < 0.000$ (Cramer's V = 0.18; Kendall's Tau-B = –0.17; $p < 0.000$).

Question Wording: *Quality of Services:* See Table 3.1. *Satisfaction:* In general, would you say you are satisfied, neither satisfied nor dissatisfied, dissatisfied with the way health care runs in your country? The value of p is indicated for Pearson's $\chi 2$ and Kendall's tau-b. Tau is generally the leading measure of association for ordinal variable (Lewis-Beck, 1995). A tau of 1.0 (–1.0) indicates a perfect positive (negative) monotonic relationship. A tau of 0.00 indicates no monotonic relationship. Although there are two tau measures in common use, tau-b and tau-c substantively, the differences between the two are small. Throughout the book tau-b is reported in order to facilitate comparison across tables.

to general political attitudes. Second, and more importantly, these analyses make clear the importance of ideology and politics in attitudes about health care in the US: in each case, general political values are strongly associated with health care system satisfaction in the US, but not in Canada.

Party Identification

Our survey asked respondents which party they identified with in general. Among Canadians, the distribution of declared party ID (after the "don't know" responses have been excluded) was as follows: 34% Liberals, 30% Conservatives, 15% NDP, 11% Bloquists, 9% Greens, and 1% other parties. The distribution among Americans who declared their party ID was 37% Democrats, 29% Republicans, and 34% Independents.[2]

What is the expected correlation between party ID and satisfaction with the health care system? There is evidence that Canadians who identify with the Liberal Party of Canada are somewhat more likely to have a favorable opinion of the health care system (Blidook 2008). However, we know that health care presents characteristics more in line with a "valence" issue in Canada. Satisfaction with the health care system is expected to be spread rather evenly across all party supporters, with the exception of the Bloc

Québécois. Quebecers who identify with the Bloc are as supportive of the principle of public health care as other Canadians are, but they are less supportive of the current organization of the Canadian health care system (Hébert 2012). The Canadian health care system treats all provinces the same, but many Bloc Québécois supporters want Quebec to be treated differently. This wish is illustrated by the following quote from the Bloc's platform *Présent pour le Québec* at the 2008 federal election: "The Bloc wants to eliminate the fiscal imbalance and eliminate the spending power that the federal government has unilaterally arrogated to itself in areas such as health care that fall under the jurisdiction of Québec."[3] In Canada, then, party ID is not expected to make a large difference in satisfaction with the health care system except for the Bloc Québécois. But the reason why Bloc supporters are less satisfied with the health care system than the supporters of other parties has less to do with differences in perception of health care issues than with disagreement about the roles of the federal and the provincial governments in health care.[4]

In the US, there is evidence that party ID is strongly correlated with divided public attitudes toward the health care system. Brewer (2005) has shown that the issue of government health insurance has been more divisive among party lines than the issues of abortion, guaranteed jobs, or school prayer (see also Baldassari and Gelman 2008). Judging by the heated partisan debates surrounding the passage of President Barack Obama's Affordable Care Act in 2010, it appears that the partisan conflict over health care has intensified recently.

As far as the direction of the correlation between party ID and satisfaction, in Canada it is hypothesized that Bloc supporters will be more dissatisfied with the health care system than supporters of other parties. In the US it is hypothesized that Republican identifiers will support their health care system more than Democratic identifiers. In view of the partisan polarization on this issue in the US, it is hypothesized that the correlation between party ID and satisfaction with the health care system will be stronger in the US than in Canada.

Results are shown in Table 4.2. As hypothesized, satisfaction is correlated with party ID in the US. More Republican identifiers are satisfied (47%) than dissatisfied (33%) and more Democratic identifiers are dissatisfied (40%) than satisfied (37%). Note that the proportion of satisfied Americans is the same for Independents (37%) as for Democrats. In Canada, there are many more satisfied than dissatisfied Canadians among Conservative, Liberal, New Democratic, and Green supporters. Bloc supporters are the exception as hypothesized, with 46% dissatisfied and 31% satisfied with the health care system. When Bloquists are removed, the correlation between partisan ID and satisfaction with the health care system in Canada totally disappears.

In the US, bivariate correlations in Table 4.2 can be interpreted causally in two distinct ways. On the one hand, party ID could be considered as the independent variable, "causing" citizens' attitudes toward health care.

Table 4.2 Party ID and Satisfaction with the Health Care System

	Canada				US		
	Very/Fairly Dissatisfied	Neither Satisfied nor Dissatisfied	Fairly/Very Satisfied		Very/Fairly Dissatisfied	Neither Satisfied nor Dissatisfied	Fairly/Very Satisfied
Conservative	22	16	62	Republican	33	20	47
Liberal	20	16	64	Democrat	40	23	37
NDP	28	13	59	Independent	42	20	37
Bloquist	46	23	31	Libertarian	60	5	35
Green	17	19	64				
Other/it varies	23	20	57	Other	40	20	40
None	27	25	48	Don't know	39	38	23

Notes: Sample sizes are 3,522 and 3,542 for Canada and the US, respectively. Data are weighted. *Canada:* $\chi 2 = 152.6$ with 12 df; $p < 0.000$ (Cramer's V = 0.15; Kendall's Tau-B = –0.10; $p < 0.000$). *US:* $\chi 2 = 85.2$ with 10 df; $p < 0.000$ (Cramer's V = 0.11; Kendall's Tau-B = –0.08; $p < 0.000$).

Question Wording: *Canadian Sample:* Generally speaking, do you usually think of yourself as a Liberal, Conservative, New Democrat, Bloquist, or what? *American Sample:* Generally speaking, do you usually think of yourself as a Democrat, a Republican, an Independent, or what?

In this formulation, party ID constitutes a "perceptual screen" (Campbell et al. 1960) or an "information shortcut" (Sniderman, Brody, and Tetlock 1991; Popkin 1991) through which citizens can form an opinion about the health care system. Republican Party supporters are satisfied with the current private market-based health care system based on their knowledge that it is the system that their preferred party is advocating. Democrats are dissatisfied with the current private market–based health care system based on their knowledge that their preferred party wants to change it into a different system.

There is an alternative formulation of party ID as a dependent variable, determined by citizens' satisfaction toward health care. According to this formulation, citizens will support the party with the health care policy program closest to their own preferred position. Americans who prefer a private market–based health care system will be more likely to identify with the Republican Party as a result, while Americans who prefer a public health care system will be more likely to identify with the Democratic Party as a result. In other words, party ID is a consequence rather than a cause of citizens' satisfaction with health care.

The bivariate association of Table 4.2 cannot determine which causal pathway is correct. To test the idea that party ID may be influenced by satisfaction, we have run a multivariate linear regression model for the impact of satisfaction on party ID, controlling for the impact of citizens' attitudes toward private market–based health care as a symbol of what it means to be American. Party ID is coded +1 for Democrats, 0 for Independents, and –1 for Republicans. The coefficients for both variables are positive by hypothesis. The results clearly indicate that citizens' symbolic attitudes have a strong statistical impact on party ID, whereas satisfaction has no impact. We will return to citizens' symbolic attitudes toward their health care system later in the chapter. We will see in the next chapter that citizens' symbolic attitudes have a strong statistical impact on satisfaction even after controlling for the effect of many other variables. Clearly, citizens' symbolic values are an antecedent variable influencing both satisfaction and party ID in such a way that no variation is left in party ID to be independently explained by satisfaction. By contrast, the multivariate results in Chapter 5 show that party ID has a significant independent impact on satisfaction in the US (Table 5.2). The data appear to support the interpretation of party ID as a causal factor that shapes citizens satisfaction with the health care system, but not the reverse interpretation of party ID as a consequence of satisfaction with the health care system.

Left-Right (Liberal-Conservative) Ideology

Survey respondents were asked to place themselves on a six-point left-right scale in Canada, and on a similar six-point liberal-conservative scale in the US. A 0 value on the scale denotes a strong left/liberal ideology, a value of

Table 4.3 Left-Right (Liberal-Conservative) Ideology

	Canada	US
Left/liberal	11	17
Center-left	15	18
Center	33	10
Center-right	26	28
Right/conservative	15	28

Notes: Sample sizes are 3,522 and 3,542 for Canada and the US, respectively. Data are weighted.

$\chi 2 = 620.5$ with 4 df; $p < 0.000$ (Cramer's V = 0.30; Kendall's Tau-B = 0.07; $p < 0.000$).

Question Wording: *Canadian Sample:* In politics people sometimes talk of being on the left or the right. Where would you place yourself on a left-right scale? *American Sample:* In politics people sometimes talk of being liberal or conservative. Where would you place yourself on a liberal-conservative scale?

1 denotes a center-left ideology. A value of 4 on the scale denotes a center-right ideology and a value of 5 denotes a firm right/conservative ideology. The values 2 and 3 represent a "centrist" position (or "neither left nor right") for the purposes of our analysis (Table 4.3).

Many more Canadians (33%) position themselves as neither left nor right on the scale than Americans (10%), in line with the idea that Canadian voters (and parties) are generally more centrist. Canadians who declare a position on the left or on the right of the scale are split 39% left and 61% right (excluding the center from the calculation). The numbers in the US are 39% liberals versus 61% conservatives. These results are consistent with previous evidence about left-right placement in Canada (Gibbins and Nevitte 1985; Gidengil et al. 2004; Cochrane 2010) and liberal/conservative placement in the US (Jacoby 2009).[5]

What correlation between left-right ideological self-placement and satisfaction with the health care system should be expected? Let us look at the direction of the correlation first. In general, the substantive meaning of left/liberal is associated with state intervention, and the substantive meaning of right/conservative is associated with freedom from the state. The Canadian health care system being characterized by state intervention, it is hypothesized that Canadians who place themselves on the left or the center-left tend to be more satisfied than dissatisfied with their public health care system, whereas Canadians who identify with the right or the center-right tend to be more dissatisfied than satisfied. The US health care system being characterized by freedom from state intervention, it is hypothesized that Americans who identify with liberalism tend to be dissatisfied rather than satisfied with the private health care system of the US. Conversely, Americans who identify with conservatism

Table 4.4 Left-Right Ideology and Satisfaction with the Health Care System

	Canada			US		
	Very/ Fairly Dissatisfied	Neither Satisfied nor Dissatisfied	Fairly/ Very Satisfied	Very/ Fairly Dissatisfied	Neither Satisfied nor Dissatisfied	Fairly/ Very Satisfied
Left/liberal	21	17	61	52	18	30
Center-left	24	17	59	42	21	37
Center	29	19	52	41	35	24
Center-right	27	21	53	35	23	42
Right/ conservative	21	16	63	34	20	47

Notes: Sample sizes are 3,522 and 3,542 for Canada and the US, respectively. Data are weighted. *Canada:* $\chi 2 = 29.6$ with 8 df; $p < 0.000$ (Cramer's V = 0.07; Kendall's Tau-B = 0.00; $p < 0.992$). *US:* $\chi 2 = 127.4$ with 8 df; $p < 0.000$ (Cramer's V = 0.13; Kendall's Tau-B = 0.12; $p < 0.000$).

tend to be satisfied with their health care system. As far as the strength of the correlation is concerned, based on our earlier observation that the debate on health care is more ideologically-oriented in the US, the correlation between left-right self-placement and satisfaction with the health care system is expected to be stronger in this country. In Canada, left-right ideology is not expected to be a factor influencing satisfaction with the health care system.

Table 4.4 displays the data. It can be seen that the US part of the hypothesis is supported by the data. Among Americans declaring that they are liberals, only 30% are satisfied (and 52% dissatisfied) with their health care system, and among those declaring that they are conservatives, the split is 47% satisfied versus 34% dissatisfied. The relationship between satisfaction with the health care system and liberal-conservative ideology is statistically significant and positive (tau-b of 0.12, $p < 0.00$).

Our Canadian hypothesis is supported as well: Canadians are satisfied with their health care system whether they are from the left or from the right. The relationship is practically non-existent in Canada (tau-b of 0.00). As can be seen, there are not that many more Canadians positioned on the right who are satisfied with their health care system (63%) than Canadians declaring that they are on the left (61%). Left-right ideology appears to be related to satisfaction with the health care system in the US, but not in Canada.

Individualism and Attitude About the Role of Government

Our survey asked respondents six questions that were used to construct an individualism-collectivism scale going from one (extreme individualistic) to five (extreme collectivist). (Full question wordings are provided in the Appendix.) The survey also asked respondents to place themselves on a five-point scale measuring their attitude toward the role of government in general. The value 1 on the scale coincides with the statement that the "government should let each person get ahead on his own" (small role of government), and the value 5 coincides with the statement that the "government should see to it that every person has a job" (large role of government).

There is a debate about whether and to what extent Americans are more individualistic and private market oriented while Canadians are more collectivist and more state oriented. According to Lipset's (1990) "defining moment" interpretation, the political cultures of the two countries were set on two different paths by the American Revolution and the Loyalist migration to Canada that followed. The Loyalist migration in Canada set the stage for a "collectivist/statist" political culture characterized by a willingness to use the state to protect citizens from the effects of economic inequality, an emphasis on achieving equality of conditions, and by popular deference toward the governing elite. The fact that the US achieved independence by an act of war set American political culture on an "individualistic" course that emphasized suspicion of the state, achieving equality of opportunity rather than equality of conditions, and egalitarianism. More recently, Adams (2003) has also argued that Americans are exceptionally individualistic while Canadians retain collectivist values that resemble those found in Western Europe.

Grabb and Curtis (2005, 168) find little support for Lipset's claim of a collectivist/statist political culture in Canada from the historical record. They argue that the typical pattern in Canada was much the same as that found in the US. From recent World Values Survey data, they find no significant differences in Americans' and Canadians' individualist attitudes today. On the other hand, they find some small differences in attitudes toward the role of the state (see Perlin 1997 for a similar diagnosis).

Table 4.5 displays the placement of Americans and Canadians on the individualism-collectivism scale, based on our own more recent data. Results appear to support Grabb and Curtis' interpretation that Americans'

Table 4.5 Collectivism-Individualism Scale

	Canada	US
Extreme collectivist	12	19
Collectivist	26	22
Neither collectivist nor individualist	43	37
Individualist	16	15
Extreme individualist	3	6

Notes: Sample sizes are 3,522 and 3,542 for Canada and the US, respectively. Data are weighted. $\chi 2 = 120.9$ with 4 df; $p < 0.000$ (Cramer's V = 0.13; Kendall's Tau-B = 0.03; $p < 0.02$). Question wording provided in the Appendix.

Table 4.6 Role of Government Scale

	Canada	US
1. See that every person has a job	14	11
2	18	16
3	46	40
4	13	17
5. Let each person get ahead on his own	9	16

Notes: Sample sizes are 3,522 and 3,542 for Canada and the US, respectively. Data are weighted. $\chi2 = 129.8$ with 4 df; $p < 0.000$ (Cramer's $V = 0.14$; Kendall's Tau-B $= 0.11$; $p < 0.000$).

Question Wording: Some people say that the government in Ottawa (in Washington) should see to it that every person has a job and a good standard of living. Other people say that the government should just let each person get ahead on his own. And of course other people have opinions somewhere in between.

and Canadians' individualist attitudes are similar. There is certainly considerable overlap in Americans' and Canadians' positions, although there are more extreme individualists and extreme collectivists among Americans than among Canadians.[6]

Table 4.6 compares Americans' and Canadians' views of the role of government. Americans are more likely than Canadians to agree that government should "let each person get ahead on his own" (33% versus 22% when scores of four and five are added). They are also less likely than Canadians to agree that "government should see to it that every person has a job" (27% versus 32% when scores of one and two are added). It can be seen that Americans' and Canadians' attitudes toward the role of government differ more than their collectivist/statist political cultures. Still, these differences are now huge and, as we will see, pale in comparison to Americans' and Canadians' views about health care.[7]

It is hypothesized that individualistic Americans tend to be satisfied with their health care system more often than collectivist Americans. On the other hand, it is hypothesized that Canadians' level of satisfaction with their health care system does not correlate with their placement on the individualist-collectivist scale. As Table 4.7 shows, the hypothesis is supported by the data in the US. Individualist Americans are significantly more satisfied (51%) than dissatisfied (33%) with their health care system, and collectivist Americans are significantly more dissatisfied (59%) than satisfied (23%) with their health care system (significant tau-b of 0.16 for the US). The hypothesis of no correlation is also supported by the data in Canada. Canadians are satisfied with the health care system irrespective of whether they are individualists or collectivists (tau-b of 0.00).

What is the expected impact of attitudes on the role of government on satisfaction with the health care system? As far as the direction of the impact

Table 4.7 Individualism and Satisfaction with the Health Care System

	Canada			US		
	Very/Fairly Dissatisfied	Neither Satisfied nor Dissatisfied	Fairly/ Very Satisfied	Very/Fairly Dissatisfied	Neither Satisfied nor Dissatisfied	Fairly/ Very Satisfied
Extreme collectivist	29	16	55	59	18	23
Collectivist	26	17	57	40	21	39
Neither collectivist nor individualist	23	23	55	32	28	40
Individualist	27	15	58	34	18	48
Extreme individualist	36	10	54	33	15	51

Notes: Sample sizes are 3,522 and 3,542 for Canada and the US, respectively. Data are weighted.
Canada: $\chi 2 = 37.9$ with 8 df; $p < 0.000$ (Cramer's V = 0.07; Kendall's Tau-B = 0.00; $p < 0.907$).
US: $\chi 2 = 189.5$ with 8 df; $p < 0.000$ (Cramer's V = 0.16; Kendall's Tau-B = 0.16; $p < 0.000$).

goes, in Canada, where the role of government is large, it is hypothesized that people who agree that "government should see to it that every person has a job" are more satisfied with their health care system than people who agree that "government should let each person get ahead on his own." In the US, where the role of government is more limited, it is hypothesized that people who believe in a limited role of government are more satisfied with their health care system, whereas those who believe in an extended role of government are less satisfied with their health care system. As far as the strength of the impact goes, it is hypothesized that their attitudes about the role of government has no polarizing effect on their satisfaction with the health care system. By contrast, it is hypothesized that Americans' attitudes toward the role of government will have a polarizing effect on their satisfaction with the health care system.

Results are displayed in Table 4.8, and our hypothesis is supported by the US data. Americans who strongly agree that government should let each person get ahead on his own are more satisfied than dissatisfied with their health care system (52% to 32%). Dissatisfaction with their health care system occurs significantly more frequently among Americans who strongly agree that "government should see to it that every person has a job" (54% versus 31%). The relationship is statistically significant at $p < 0.00$ (tau-b of 0.13). In the Canadian case, the relationship is much weaker than in the US (tau-b of 0.04) and it is only significant at $p < 0.02$.

Table 4.8 View on the Role of Government and Satisfaction with the Health Care System

	Canada			US		
	Very/Fairly Dissatisfied	Neither Satisfied nor Dissatisfied	Fairly/ Very Satisfied	Very/Fairly Dissatisfied	Neither Satisfied nor Dissatisfied	Fairly/ Very Satisfied
1. See that every person has a job	34	18	48	54	14	31
2	26	15	59	44	24	32
3	22	21	56	37	28	35
4	24	18	58	36	19	45
5. Let each person get ahead on his own	29	13	58	32	17	52

Notes: Sample sizes are 3,522 and 3,542 for Canada and the US, respectively. Data are weighted.
Canada: $\chi 2 = 44.3$ with 8 df; $p < 0.000$ (Cramer's V = 0.08; Kendall's Tau-B = 0.04; $p < 0.013$).
US: $\chi 2 = 127.1$ with 8 df; $p < 0.000$ (Cramer's V = 0.13; Kendall's Tau-B = 0.13; $p < 0.000$).

POLITICAL VALUES AND ATTITUDES RELATED TO HEALTH CARE

As we have just seen, there is no link between Canadians' levels of satisfaction with their health care system and their attitudes toward individualism, left-right ideology, or the role of the government. Now we turn to attitudes more directly related to health care. To what extent do attitudes about the nature of health care correlate with satisfaction with the health care system?

Our survey asked respondents to place themselves on a five-point "access to health care" scale. Scores one and two on the scale are for respondents who place themselves at or near the statement, "We must do everything to protect universal access to health care regardless of ability to pay." Scores four and five are for those who place themselves at or near the statement, "Ensuring universal access regardless of ability to pay is simply too costly." Respondents who take a position between these extremes receive a score of three. The survey also asked respondents to place themselves on a similar five-point "health insurance" scale where support and near support for the statement, "We must do everything we can to protect government insurance for all expenses for everyone" is scored one and two, respectively, at one extreme on the scale, support and near support for the statement, "We must rely on private insurance for all expenses for everyone" is scored four and five, respectively, at the other extreme, and the position between is scored three.

As we have seen in Chapter 2, Canadian public opinion has become more supportive than American public opinion of an active role of government, especially in health care, in the last decades (see also Boychuk 2008; Hacker 1998; Maioni 1998; Perlin 1997). Surveys about Canadians' political values concerning health care have sent a clear and consistent message since they started to be administered on a regular basis in the 1990s: Canadians have demonstrated an unwavering attachment to the principles of a single-payer government health care insurance plan for all and equal access to health care, even in the face of deepening anxiety over system deterioration. A 1998 Pollara-Earnscliffe Research and Communication poll found that 91% of Canadians agreed and 9% disagreed with the notion of equal access regardless of need or ability to pay. In a 2002 Pollara poll, 87% of Canadians agreed and 11% disagreed that "universal access to health care is a Canadian core value." Polls have also shown how deeply the principle of government health care insurance for everyone is embedded within Canadian sense of values. According to a 2010 Environics Focus Canada Survey, 78% of Canadians declared that health insurance should be paid for by government rather than by the private sector (14%), largely unchanged from 2004.

In the US, polls conducted since the early 1980s have repeatedly shown that the American public is unable to agree on what type of health insurance plan they support. For example, a Washington Post/Kaiser Family Foundation/Harvard University poll conducted in the summer of 2000 revealed that 54% of registered voters favored (and 34% opposed) a national health insurance financed by taxes. But when the poll question was modified by adding a clause specifying that all Americans would obtain their health insurance from a single government plan, support fell to 38% (and opposition rose to 58%) of registered voters.

Note that unlike questions in these Pollara, Environics, and Kaiser Foundations polls, which only ask respondents to agree or disagree with a statement, the health-insurance question and the access-to-health-care questions in our survey allow respondents to pick a median response "in between" two positions. Regarding the issue of access to health care, 68% of Canadians support "universal access regardless of ability to pay," 13% support the statement that "universal access is simply too costly," while 20% place themselves "in-between" these two options (Table 4.9). Among Americans, 41% support "universal access regardless of ability to pay," 36% support the statement that "universal access is simply too costly," and 24% place themselves "in between" these two positions.

Americans' and Canadians' attitudes on the issue of who should pay for health care insurance are distributed similarly to their attitudes on the issue of access to health care (Table 4.10). Sixty-six percent of Canadians but only 42% of Americans support the idea of government insurance for everyone; 28% of Americans but only 8% of Canadians support the principle of private insurance for all. Note the comparatively high proportions of

Table 4.9 Universal or Limited Access to Health Care?

	Canada	US
1. Universal access	46	24
2	22	17
3	20	24
4	7	15
5. Simply too costly	6	21

Notes: Sample sizes are 3,522 and 3,542 for Canada and the US, respectively. Data are weighted. $\chi 2 = 553.9$ with 4 df; $p < 0.000$ (Cramer's $V = 0.30$; Kendall's Tau-B $= 0.27$; $p < 0.000$).

Question Wording: Some people say that ensuring that health care is universally available to everyone, regardless of their ability to pay, is so important that we do everything we can to protect these principles. Other people say that enduring universal access, regardless of ability to pay, is simply too costly.

Table 4.10 Government or Private Health Insurance?

	Canada	US
1. Government insurance	39	24
2	27	18
3	26	29
4	5	14
5. Private insurance	3	14

Notes: Sample sizes are 3,522 and 3,542 for Canada and the US, respectively. Data are weighted. $\chi 2 = 549.3$ with 4 df; $p < 0.000$ (Cramer's $V = 0.30$; Kendall's Tau-B $= 0.24$; $p < 0.000$). Question Wording: Some people say that there should be a government insurance plan which would cover all medical and hospital expenses for everyone. Other people say that all medical expenses should be paid by individuals, and through private insurance plans like Blue Cross.

Canadians (26%) and Americans (29%) who place themselves "in between" on the health insurance issue.

Two points can be drawn from the data of Tables 4.9 and 4.10. First, Canadians' support for universal access to health care and for public health insurance (68% and 66% respectively) is approximately twice as high as their (32%) support of a large role of government. Americans' support for universal access to health care and for public health insurance (41% and 42% respectively) is also above their support for a large role of government in general (27%)—although the gap is smaller than in Canada. More Canadians and, to a lesser extent, more Americans support a large role of government in health care than they support a large role of government in general. Although the questions are different (one asks about a change in the size of government while the other asks about support for levels of health care) and thus are difficult to compare directly, they do provide further indication that the moderate difference in Americans' and Canadians' expressed support for larger government becomes much larger when it comes to health care.[8] Second, there is a marked contrast between the widely shared core values of universal access and government insurance in Canada and the ideological divide that separates Americans' perceptions of these issues.[9]

What is the expected correlation between attitudes about the role of government in health care and satisfaction with the health care system? It is hypothesized that people who support a large role of government in health insurance and in protecting universal access to health care are more satisfied than dissatisfied with the public-oriented health care system of Canada, and more dissatisfied than satisfied with the private-oriented health care system of the US.

The hypothesis is supported by the data in both Canada and the US. Satisfaction with their health care system occurs significantly more frequently among Americans who agree that universal health care is simply too costly (49%). On the other hand, 58% of Americans who strongly agree that everything should be done to protect universal access are dissatisfied with their health care system. The correlation between attitude toward access to health care and satisfaction with the system is positive and significant (tau-b of 0.19). Among Canadians who strongly agree that everything should be done to protect universal access to health care, 60% are satisfied with their health care system. But only 37% of Canadians who strongly agree that universal access is too costly are satisfied with the health care system (Table 4.11). Contrary to

Table 4.11 Attitude about Access to Health Care and Satisfaction with the Health Care System

	Canada			US		
	Very/Fairly Dissatisfied	Neither Satisfied nor Dissatisfied	Fairly/ Very Satisfied	Very/Fairly Dissatisfied	Neither Satisfied nor Dissatisfied	Fairly/ Very Satisfied
1. Universal access	25	15	60	58	13	29
2	20	18	62	49	23	28
3	27	19	54	33	23	44
4	28	22	51	33	18	49
5. Simply too costly	46	17	37	29	22	49

Notes: Sample sizes are 3,522 and 3,542 for Canada and the US, respectively. Data are weighted.
Canada: $\chi2 = 69.7$ with 8 df; $p < 0.000$ (Cramer's V = 0.11; Kendall's Tau-B = –0.08; $p < 0.000$).
US: $\chi2 = 191.4$ with 8 df; $p < 0.000$ (Cramer's V = 0.18; Kendall's Tau-B = 0.19; $p < 0.000$).

Table 4.12 Attitude about Health Insurance and Satisfaction with the Health Care System

	Canada			US		
	Very/Fairly Dissatisfied	Neither Satisfied nor Dissatisfied	Fairly/ Very Satisfied	Very/Fairly Dissatisfied	Neither Satisfied nor Dissatisfied	Fairly/ Very Satisfied
1. Government insurance	29	15	55	56	18	27
2	20	17	63	51	19	30
3	24	20	57	36	24	39
4	30	28	42	27	20	54
5. Private insurance	37	25	39	25	17	57

Notes: Sample sizes are 3,522 and 3,542 for Canada and the US, respectively. Data are weighted.

Canada: $\chi 2$ = 53.4 with 8 df; $p < 0.000$ (Cramer's V = 0.09; Kendall's Tau-B = –0.008; $p < 0.605$).

US: $\chi 2$ = 223.9 with 8 df; $p < 0.000$ (Cramer's V = 0.19; Kendall's Tau-B = 0.22; $p < 0.000$).

the US, then, the correlation is negative (significant tau-b of –0.08) and clearly smaller. The same inverse relationships can be observed when we compare the two countries in terms of attitudes about health insurance. Among Canadians who strongly agree that government insurance plan should cover all expenses for everyone, 55% are satisfied with their health care system. But only 39% of Canadians who agree that health care expenses should be paid by individuals and by private insurance plans are satisfied with the health care system (Table 4.12). The correlation is negative but not statistically significant (tau-b of –0.01), while in the US it is positive and significant (tau-b of 0.22).

PERCEPTIONS OF HEALTH CARE AS NATIONAL SYMBOL

For the past fifteen years, Environics Focus Canada surveys have found the health care system to be at the top of the list of symbols of Canadian identity. In the 2010 Focus Canada survey, 85% of Canadians declared the health care system to be a "very important" symbol of Canadian identity, ahead of other familiar symbols as the Charter of rights and freedom (78%), the Canadian flag (73%), national parks (72%), and the national anthem (66%). By contrast, health care never appears on any list of symbols of national unity in the US.

This situation seems peculiar to Canada. Our survey asked Americans whether they agreed or disagreed with the statement that "market-based health care is part of what it means to be American." Canadian were asked whether they agree or disagreed with the statement that "universal publicly-funded health care is part of what it means to be Canadian." Table 4.13 displays the contrast between Americans' and Canadians' perceptions of how health care defines what it means to be American or Canadian. Less than half (43%) of Americans agree with the statement that "market-based health care is part of what it means to be American" versus 57% who either disagree with or are unsure of the statement. This denotes a lack of consensus on the topic in the US as opposed to a strong consensus in Canada, where 82% of the respondents agree with the statement that "universal publicly-funded health care is part of what it means to be Canadian," while only 18% either disagree with or are unsure of the statement. At the very least, these figures suggest that in people's minds a relationship between a health care model and the US is weaker than a relationship between a health care model and Canada.[10]

Our survey also asked Canadians and Americans whether they thought that their health care system was a unifying symbol of their country and its people. As Table 4.14 shows, the perceptions of Americans and Canadians toward health care as a symbol unifying their country are very different. Only 32% of Americans consider their health care system as a unifying symbol, versus 68% who don't. On the other hand, 77% of Canadians consider

Table 4.13 Part of What It Means to Be Canadian/American

	Canada	US
Strongly agree	48	14
Somewhat agree	34	29
Neither agree nor disagree	13	33
Somewhat disagree	3	11
Strongly disagree	2	13

Notes: Sample sizes are 3,522 and 3,542 for Canada and the US, respectively. Data are weighted. Question Wording: *Canadian Sample:* Universal publicly-funded health care is part of what it means to be Canadian and reflects our core values. *American Sample:* Market-based health care is part of what it means to be American and reflects our core values.

Table 4.14 Health Care as Symbol of National Unity

	Canada	US
Not a unifying symbol	23	68
Unifying symbol	77	32

Notes: Sample sizes are 3,522 and 3,542 for Canada and the US, respectively. Data are weighted. Question Wording: Do you consider the health care system as a unifying symbol of your country and its people?

Table 4.15 Health Care as Unifying Symbol of National Unity and Satisfaction with the Health Care System

	Canada			US		
	Very/Fairly Dissatisfied	Neither Satisfied nor Dissatisfied	Fairly/ Very Satisfied	Very/Fairly Dissatisfied	Neither Satisfied nor Dissatisfied	Fairly/ Very Satisfied
Not a unifying symbol	39	21	40	44	21	35
Unifying symbol	21	16	63	35	19	46

Notes: Sample sizes are 3,522 and 3,542 for Canada and the US, respectively. Data are weighted.
Canada: $\chi2 = 127.6$ with 2 df; $p < 0.000$ (Cramer's V = 0.20; Kendall's Tau-B = 0.19; $p < 0.000$).
US: $\chi2 = 35.0$ with 2 df; $p < 0.000$ (Cramer's V = 0.11; Kendall's Tau-B = 0.10; $p < 0.000$).

their health care system as a unifying symbol, against 23% who don't. The difference is not difficult to explain: Canadians, being strongly united in their support of the public health care system, are strongly inclined to consider it a symbol of national unity. But Americans cannot hold something that divides them as a symbol of national unity.[11]

In Canada, where the health care system is considered by most as a unifying symbol, it is hypothesized that perception of health care as a symbol of national unity correlates positively with satisfaction with the health care system. In the US, where health care is not a symbol of national unity, it is hypothesized that there is no correlation. The results are displayed in Table 4.15. The perception of the health care system as a symbol of national unity is positively and significantly correlated with satisfaction with the system in both countries. However the correlation is much stronger in Canada (tau-b of 0.19) than in the US (tau-b of 0.10). As Table 4.15 indicates, there are many more satisfied Canadians (63%) among those who consider health care as a unifying symbol than among those who don't (40%). The proportions of satisfied Americans who consider the health care system as a symbol of national unity is 46%, against 35% satisfied Americans who do not consider the system as a symbol of national unity.

WITHIN-COUNTRY AND ACROSS-COUNTRY VARIATIONS IN ATTITUDES TOWARD HEALTH CARE

In their thought-provoking book, Grabb and Curtis (2005) argue that North America is formed of "four societies"—English Canada (ROC, for Rest of Canada), Quebec, the American South (South), and the other states of the

Union (ROU, for Rest of Union). According to these authors, these regions, due to their peculiar historical paths, are characterized by the distinct political profiles of their populations, Quebec being the most progressive region, the US South the most conservative, and the other regions, ROC and ROU, being more moderate and more similar.

According to Grabb and Curtis, it is the exceptionalism of Quebec and the South that explains what has in previous research been attributed to national-level Canada-US differences. An assessment of the relevance of across-country differences in Americans' and Canadians' social and political attitudes ultimately depends of course on the magnitude of within-country differences in those attitudes. Therefore, in order to address Grabb and Curtis' point, we need to know how much difference in attitudes toward health care there is among regions within Canada and the US. The place to start is to look at the level of satisfaction toward the health care system in the four regions. This information is provided in Table 4.16. The results in this table are interesting on many accounts. First, they confirm, as it has been observed many times over the last fifteen years, that Quebecers are notoriously less satisfied with the performance of their health care system than the rest of Canadians are (e.g., Bélanger and Nadeau 2009). The rate of satisfaction toward the health care system is only 35% in Quebec, almost thirty points lower than the level observed in the ROC (63%). This difference is huge and is of course statistically significant (tau-b = 0.25, p = 0.00).

Perhaps more importantly, the data convincingly demonstrate that Canada-US differences are not driven by within-country variation. First,

Table 4.16 Satisfaction with the Health Care System: Quebec, Rest of Canada (ROC), Rest of the Union (ROU), South

	Very/Fairly Dissatisfied	Neither Satisfied nor Dissatisfied	Fairly/Very Satisfied
Canada	25	19	56
Quebec	41	24	35
Rest of Canada (ROC)	21	17	63
US	39	22	39
South	40	22	38
Rest of Union (ROU)	39	23	39

Notes: Sample sizes are 946 for Quebec, 2,576 for the Rest of Canada, 2,427 for the Rest of the Union, and 1,115 for the South. Data are weighted.

Quebec vs. ROC: $\chi2$ = 291.2 with 2 df; p < 0.000 (Cramer's V = 0.25; Kendall's Tau-B = –0.24; p < 0.000).

South vs. ROU: $\chi2$ = 0.43 with 2 df; p < 0.81 (Cramer's V = 0.01; Kendall's Tau-B = –0.01; p < 0.58).

Table 4.17 Role of Government Scale: Quebec, Rest of Canada (ROC), Rest of the Union (ROU), South

	Quebec	ROC	ROU	South
1. See that every person has a job	21	12	11	12
2	21	17	17	15
3	40	47	40	39
4	12	14	17	17
5. Let each person get ahead on his own	6	10	15	18

Notes: Sample sizes are 946 for Quebec, 2,576 for the Rest of Canada, 2,427 for the Rest of the Union, and 1,115 for the South. Data are weighted.

Quebec vs. ROC: $\chi 2 = 59.2$ with 4 df; $p < 0.000$ (Cramer's V = 0.13; Kendall's Tau-B = –0.10; $p < 0.000$).

South vs. ROU: $\chi 2 = 7.6$ with 2 df; $p < 0.11$ (Cramer's V = 0.05; Kendall's Tau-B = 0.02; $p < 0.20$).

there is virtually no difference in the level of satisfaction toward the health care system between the South and the other American states (tau-b = –0.01, p = 0.58). Second, the gap in the level of satisfaction is even higher between the ROC and the ROU (twenty-four percentage points, 63% vs. 39%)[12] than between Canada and the US as a whole (seventeen percentage points). Contrary to Grabb and Curtis' prediction, the exclusion of the "problematic" regions from the analyses, Quebec and the South, does not decrease but actually increases the observed Canada-US differences.

How can we explain this result? Why is Quebec so different? Grabb and Curtis' contention is that Quebec is the most progressive region of North America. This hypothesis seems confirmed by the data displayed in Table 4.17. Quebecers are indeed more likely than English Canadians (ROC), Southerners, or other Americans (ROU) to agree that government should see to it that every person has a job (42% versus 29%, 28%, and 27% when scores of one and two are added). The data also show that the minor differences observed between Canada and the US concerning the role of government (see Table 4.6) tend to disappear when Quebec's exceptionalism is taken into account. But these results do not explain why Quebecers are so dissatisfied with their health care system. Pro-government attitudes, like those more widely shared in Quebec, are expected to be positively, not negatively, linked to satisfaction toward the health care system in Canada. According to this reasoning, the level of satisfaction should be higher, not lower, in Quebec.

Another factor that could explain the apparent Quebec anomaly could be that the population of this province does not share the same values about the health care system as other Canadians do. The data in Table 4.18 show that this is not the case. The minor differences between Quebec and the ROC on

Table 4.18 Universal or Limited Access: Quebec, Rest of Canada (ROC), Rest of the Union (ROU), South

	Quebec	ROC	ROU	South
1. Universal access	42	47	23	24
2	21	23	17	13
3	21	17	26	25
4	8	7	14	13
5. Simply too costly	8	6	20	25

Notes: Sample sizes are 946 for Quebec, 2,576 for the Rest of Canada, 2,427 for the Rest of the Union, and 1,115 for the South. Data are weighted.

Quebec vs. ROC: $\chi 2 = 31.7$ with 4 df; $p < 0.000$ (Cramer's V = 0.10; Kendall's Tau-B = .08; $p < 0.000$).

South vs. ROU: $\chi 2 = 13.0$ with 4 df; $p < 0.01$ (Cramer's V = 0.07; Kendall's Tau-B = –0.00; $p < 0.87$).

the principle of universal accessibility of health care (63% versus 70% when values 1 and 2 are added) pale in comparison with the large gap between Canadians and Americans in general on this question. The conclusion is clear. Quebecers and Canadians share basically the same values about the health care system.[13] A Commission established by the Quebec government in the late 1990s to address the concerns of Quebecers concluded the same way and tabled recommendations essentially aimed at fixing problems with the existing health care system.[14] The gap between Canadians and Quebecers in terms of their level of satisfaction toward the health system is to be found elsewhere.

The solution to the Quebec puzzle is perhaps quite simple after all. Previous research has shown that Quebecers are particularly disappointed with the performance of their health care system since the mid-1990s, when their provincial government simultaneously introduced a major reform of the system while making drastic cuts to balance its budget. Since then, Quebecers have voiced deep dissatisfaction about a series of problems including waiting time lists and shortage of medical staff. One figure is particularly telling. While only 12% of Canadians outside Quebec reported having experienced difficulties in finding a regular doctor at the time of the survey (2011), the same proportion climbed to 26% in Quebec.[15] A common complaint in Quebec concerns wait times. An item of our questionnaire shows this aspect of Quebecers' "malaise" toward their health care system. No less than 62% of Quebecers in our sample answered yes to the question, "Over the past two years, have you or a member of your family had to wait longer than you thought was reasonable to get family health care services?" The same proportion is significantly lower at 46% in the rest of Canada (tau-b = 0.13, $p < 0.00$). Health care, not surprisingly, has become a recurrent electoral theme in Quebec over the last decade (Bélanger and Nadeau 2009; Nadeau and Bélanger 2013) with the opposition parties of the moment (and sometimes the media as well) regularly bringing to the fore what they describe as the failures of the health care system in Quebec. All this has contributed to create a widespread sense of dissatisfaction in Quebec toward the performance of the health care system. The most recent comparative study published by the Commonwealth Fund (2014) continues to confirm that among Canadians, Quebecers are the most dissatisfied about the performance of their health care system (see Breton 2014).

The findings for Quebec are a powerful reminder that a key determinant of satisfaction toward the health care system, either in general or about a specific aspect of it, lies in its performance. True, as previously shown, Quebecers have different attitudes toward the health care system because they don't like federal incursion into provincial matters, but their high level of dissatisfaction documented in this section is mainly due to a system that is made worse by provincial decisions. The attitudes of Canadians and Americans toward their health care systems are performance-responsive. Canadians are dissatisfied with wait times because they are longer in their country. Americans are concerned about the affordability of care because it is not universally available at a low cost in their own country. And Quebecers, even if they are more progressive than other North Americans and are as fond of Medicare as other Canadians, express a high level of dissatisfaction toward their health care system because they think that its performance is poorer than elsewhere in Canada.

CONCLUSION

Our findings show that Americans' general political values and attitudes are somewhat more polarized than is the case for Canadians. More importantly, these political attitudes are strongly correlated with their divided satisfaction with their health care system, which is not the case in Canada. Furthermore, Canadians have consensual values and attitudes about their health care system, and those consensual values are reflected in their like-minded satisfaction with it. Ideological values and attitudes directly related to health care are also correlated with satisfaction with the health care system in both countries. But in the US, divided opinions about health insurance and access to health care appear to have a polarizing impact on satisfaction with the health care system; in Canada, consensual opinions on these variables appear to have a unifying impact on satisfaction with the health care system. Finally, the perception of health care as a symbol of national unity appears to have a unifying effect on satisfaction with the health care system in Canada. A similar effect fails to materialize in the US due to the absence of perception of health care as a unifying symbol.

The cross-national findings in this chapter shed additional light on three important questions that are relevant to any comparative analysis of Canada and the US. First, to what extent are American and Canadian political attitudes different? Are the regional differences within each country more significant than aggregate differences between Canada and the US as Grabb and Curtis (2005) suggest? Specifically, is the country of origin statistically significant in determining public preferences for public vs. private health insurance or universal vs. limited access to health care? The bivariate analyses of this chapter strongly suggest that, to the extent that cross-country differences are more important than within-country differences, it can be said definitely that Canadians and Americans have different attitudes toward health care.

Second, are Americans' and Canadians' public opinions about health care converging or diverging? As mentioned earlier in the chapter, there is evidence to suggest that public opinions in Canada and the US are becoming more similar to one another in many policy areas (Grabb and Curtis 2005; Perlin 2007). However true the suggestion of convergent American and Canadian policy opinions might be in general, it appears less convincing in relation with satisfaction with the health care system today. As the chapter demonstrates, health care is a "valence" issue in Canada, and the peculiar symbolic attachment of Canadians to their health care system seems to contribute to an increased level of satisfaction with that system. By contrast, health care has been a "positional" issue in the US for quite some time now, and this is associated with even more divided attitudes on satisfaction with the health care system than many other policy issues among Americans today.

Third, are the differences in Americans' and Canadians' satisfaction with health care concentrated more at the elite or at the mass level? We believe it would be a mistake to interpret differences in Americans' and Canadians' levels of satisfaction with their health care systems as being entirely explained away by distinct American and Canadian "cultures." The evidence in this chapter about the impact of party identification on public opinion, especially in the US, appears to support another interpretation which emphasizes the differences in the attitudes and preferences of American and Canadian governing elites toward their health care systems. Important research on the relationship between opinion and policy has highlighted that government policies do not simply respond to the demands of the mass public but also shape them to some extent, both in the US and in Canada (Margolis and Mauser 1992; Pétry and Mendelsohn 2004; Bélanger and Pétry 2005). The way in which the American and Canadian elites frame the debate about the health care issue is clearly reflected in mass opinion. This insight, as well as others from this chapter and the one before, will inform our model of opinion formation that we will now develop and test in Chapter 5.

NOTES

1. The difference between both countries is substantial and statistically significant (tau-b = –0.17, $p < 0.00$).
2. The Conservative Party's share of the popular vote was 38% in the 2008 election and 40% in the 2011 election, and the Liberal Party's share of the popular vote was 26% in 2008 and 19% in 2011. Liberal Party identifiers are overrepresented in the Canadian sample at the expense of Conservative identifiers. According to a 2010 Gallup poll, among Americans ready to declare their party ID, there were 40% Independents, 31% Democrats, and 27% Republicans. Democratic Party identifiers are overrepresented in the American sample at the expense of Independents.
3. The platform is found on the www.poltext.org website at www.poltext.org/sites/poltext.org/files/plateformes/can2008bloc_plt_eng._14112008_164107.pdf
4. Although we do not have survey data to verify this, we can safely speculate that the correlation between party ID and satisfaction observed among Bloc supporters is a spurious side effect of the strong statistical impact of an antecedent variable on both party ID and satisfaction: support for Quebec sovereignty.
5. This result must be interpreted with caution given the different formulations and meanings of this question in the US and Canada. More suitable items will be examined later in this section to compare Americans' and Canadians' basic political attitudes.
6. The difference between both countries is small and not significant at the 0.01 level (tau-b = –0.03, $p < 0.02$).
7. The difference between both countries is significant at the 0.00 level (tau-b = 0.11); the coding of the variable means that Americans tend to adopt more systematically the values near the "let each person get ahead on his own" pole.
8. The tau-b measuring the difference across both countries is 0.11 for the general question about government's role and 0.27 ($p < 0.00$) for the specific item about health care.
9. The difference between both countries for the insurance question is also strongly significant (tau-b = 0.24, $p < 0.00$).
10. The differences across both countries are substantial and significant (tau-b = 0.41, $p < 0.00$).
11. The differences across both countries are also substantial and significant (tau-b = –0.46, $p < 0.00$).
12. Tau-b = 0.23, $p < 0.00$.
13. Results for the other variables (government versus private insurance; health care as a national symbol) are largely similar.
14. The Commission was headed by Michel Clair, a former Health Minister in Quebec (Clair 2001). Tellingly, another Commission headed by another former Health Minister, Claude Castonguay, was set up by the Quebec government in the mid-2000s to inquire again about the problems of the health care system of the province. The Commission tabled a report (Castonguay 2008) including recommendations for opening the door to a greater role of the private sector in health care delivery. This part of the report, though, was adopted under division; not surprisingly, the report was ignored by the provincial government. Even more revealing is the fact that Claude Castonguay (Castonguay 2012) later backtracked on his recommendation concerning a larger role for the private sector in the health care system, on the grounds that public opinion in Quebec was opposed to this idea.

15. Source: HRSDC calculations based on Statistics Canada. *Health indicator profile, annual estimates, by age group and sex, Canada, provinces, territories, health regions (2011 boundaries) and peer group* (CANSIM table 105–0501). Ottawa: Statistics Canada, 2012. These figures are quite close to the results observed in our own survey (12% versus 28%; tau-b = 0.19, $p < 0.00$). Quebecers are also significantly more inclined to think that there is a shortage of nurses than other Canadians (89% versus 75%; tau-b = 0.15, $p < 0.00$). Our data also show that Quebecers have more negative opinions than other Canadians about the quality of the medical care they have received, the risks of not getting needed care in the future, and the evolution of the quality of health care in the past two years.

5 An Explanatory Model of Satisfaction about Health Care

Given the importance of health care policy not just in the United States and Canada but across the developed world, it is striking that there are so few studies of the determinants of individuals' opinions about the health care system. The same is not true of other major policy domains, after all—there are vast literatures on the structure of attitudes on redistributive policy, on macroeconomic policy, and on foreign affairs, for instance. But the literature has thus far spent little time building what we might call a "standard" model of health care policy attitudes.

One possible explanation for this state of affairs points to the episodic interest of public opinion researchers toward this policy domain—it really only rises to the fore around debates on health care reform in the US (Marmor 1993), or in the face of rising dissatisfaction toward the functioning of the Canadian health care system at the end of the 1990s and at the beginning of the 2000s (Mendelsohn 2002). The large and persistent role of the economy in electoral campaigns in Canada (Nadeau and Blais 1995; Nadeau, Bélanger, and Jérôme 2012) and the US (Vavreck 2009) could also explain this situation—health care may be less salient, for researchers at least, when other major policy domains are so clearly important.

It is high time that those interested in health care focus on the structure of health care–related attitudes, then. This chapter aims to fill this gap by identifying—in a multivariate framework—the factors that explain the degree of satisfaction of both Americans and Canadians toward their respective health care system. The objective is to develop a model of opinion toward health care that will enable us to compare opinion formation in these two countries. Most of the materials in this chapter have already been examined in a descriptive fashion, in Chapters 3 and 4. The purpose of the present chapter is to establish the specific contribution of each of these factors when pitted against each other in multivariate models.

We will begin first by briefly outlining the current state of the literature on the determinants of individual-level opinion on health care. A list of our main expectations will then be presented. Next, the empirical models to be used will be explained. Finally, the results and their implications will be presented and discussed.

INDIVIDUAL-LEVEL DETERMINANTS OF OPINIONS ON HEALTH CARE

Given its nature and importance, political scientists have devoted relatively little attention to the evolution of public opinion on health care. There are however some notable exceptions (see especially Blendon and Taylor 1989; Blidook 2008; Gelman, Lee, and Ghitza 2010; Jacobs 2008; Soroka 2007; Soroka and Lim 2003; Soroka and Fournier 2011). For example, the studies of the Commonwealth Fund International (see Blendon et al. 2002; Soroka, Maioni, and Martin 2013) show that public opinion on health care has evolved differently in Canada than in the US for about twenty years. On the one hand, the satisfaction of Canadians toward their health care system, largely higher than in the US, dropped in the late 1990s and early 2000s before recovering thereafter. On the other hand, the opinion of Americans has been much more stable. No event similar to the budgetary cutbacks in Canada seems to have changed Americans' perceptions on health care, at least until the present day.

Studies that have sought to identify the individual-level determinants of satisfaction with one's health care system are quite rare, and those that have tried to do so in a comparative perspective are virtually nonexistent. Most of these studies have been published in public health journals. For example, Schlesinger and Lee (1993) found that individuals' opinions on health depend on the nature of their experience with the health care system and their political and ideological preferences. Blendon and Taylor (1989) have shown with bivariate analyses that satisfaction toward the health care system in the US was strongly tied to race, socioeconomic status, and the health care coverage of the individual, with blacks, low-income individuals, and those generally unable to obtain certain services being less satisfied with their health care system and wanting a Canadian-style system. In a more recent study of five countries (Canada, the US, Australia, New Zealand, and the UK) Blendon and his coauthors (2002) have also noted, still using tabular analyses, that dissatisfaction toward one's health care system was particularly pronounced among those with a low income and those who have had difficulty in obtaining care.

Studies systematically comparing the determinants of opinion toward health care in the US and Canada using micro-level data are rare, but not nonexistent. Two of them used a study carried out on 3,505 Canadians and 5,813 Americans between November 2002 and March 2003 (Lasser, Himmelstein, and Woolhandler 2006; Sanmartin et al. 2006). These studies have concluded that the disparities in access to health care were more pronounced in the US than in Canada and that blacks and less affluent individuals in the US were particularly susceptible to be deprived of care and even more inclined to express a lower level of satisfaction with the functioning of the health care system.

Canadian studies on satisfaction toward the health care system have pointed out significant regional differences on this topic. Blidook (2008) has noted dissatisfaction among Quebec respondents toward their health care system and Bélanger and Nadeau (2009) have observed that this issue mattered a lot in the electoral defeat of the incumbent government in Quebec in 2003. Dissatisfaction among residents of western Canadian provinces has also been noted (Blidook 2008), a phenomenon that could be explained by clashes between certain provinces (notably Alberta) and the federal government with regard to the partial privatization of health care.

Socioeconomic disparities seem to have little impact on Canadians' opinions toward their health care system. Work by Blidook (2008) and especially that of Maioni and Martin (2004) and Soroka et al. (2013) have highlighted the importance of two types of factors that seem to weigh more on these opinions: partisan identification and the quality of care received. Blidook (2008) showed that respondents who identified with the Liberal Party of Canada were more likely to have a favorable opinion on the health care system—a result, however, that was not borne out by our own descriptive analysis in Chapter 4. Soroka et al. (2013) highlighted the decisive impact of individuals' direct experience on the evaluation of the performance of their health care system. Using an innovative approach, these authors distinguish between the retrospective evaluations of respondents, which are founded on information about the quality of care received in the past, and their prospective evaluations, which are based on their degree of confidence regarding their access to quality health care in the future, and show that these types of perceptions have a significant influence on Canadians' opinions regarding the performance of their health care system. As was seen in Chapter 3, most of these findings are confirmed in the descriptive analysis of our own data.

The rather sizeable impact of these performance variables in Soroka et al.'s (2013) study, combined with the evolution of greater satisfaction with the health care system in Canada than in the US, allows us to propose that the question of health care could present characteristics more in line with a "valence" issue in Canada, which is not the case in the US, where it seems to take on more characteristics of a "positional" issue (on this general distinction between issue types, see Stokes 1963). Canada's universal health care system is perceived by a large number of Canadians as being not only superior to other systems but also a symbol of Canadian identity (Mendelsohn 2002; Nadeau, Pétry, and Bélanger 2010; see also Chapter 4). In this sense, it is less the principles governing the organization of the system that Canadians will question than its level of performance as measured by indicators such as cost, quality, and access.

The nature of the debate over health care is more of an ideological one in the US, where it is the nature of the system itself that is at the center of debates (Marmor 1993; Jacobs and Shapiro 2000; Jacobs 2008; see also Chapter 4). The opposition between advocates of a market-centered approach with freedom of choice and those who call for more state action and implementation of policies to ensure equal access cuts the partisan (i.e., between Democrats and Republicans) and ideological (i.e., between liberals and conservatives) divides much more prominently than in Canada. Therefore it is reasonable to expect that partisan and ideological considerations will have a larger influence on Americans' opinions than those of Canadians regarding their own health care system, as already hinted at in our previous chapter.

THEORETICAL EXPECTATIONS

What can we learn from previous studies on individual-level determinants of opinions on health care, and how can these lessons help formulate more precise expectations about the explanatory factors in the US and Canada? A first observation concerns the dependent variable. Two variables have caught the attention of researchers: satisfaction toward the functioning of the health care system and opinions about the desirability of reform. These two variables are often used interchangeably, and the expectations regarding one are often stretched to fit the other. For example, in the case of the US, the typical study will tend to show that low-income individuals are both less satisfied with the current system and more inclined to want reform. In the current chapter we strictly focus on the first dependent variable, that of the respondents' satisfaction toward their own health care system. The other dependent variable, that of the extent of reforms that respondents would like to see being implemented, will be examined later, in Chapter 7.

In light of the results from Chapters 3 and 4, and of previous studies on the determinants of individual opinions—notably those on the effects of factual information, on decision-making shortcuts that make up for factual information, and on priming and framing (see especially Sniderman, Brody, and Tetlock 1991; Zaller 1992; Entman 2004; Nadeau et al. 2008; Nadeau et al. 2010)—we can express two core hypotheses to be tested in the remainder of this chapter.

First, given the larger socioeconomic disparities in the US with regard to access to care, it is expected that socioeconomic variables will have a more important impact on satisfaction toward the health care system in the US than in Canada. This issue about accessibility brings to the fore the question of coverage. In Canada, the question is almost a non-issue. In the US, quite to the contrary, accessibility to good health care for many depends crucially on the quality of the coverage offered through ones' insurance plan (see Chapter 3). To capture the impact of this key variable in spite of the complexities of the insurance schemes in the US, we use a variable asking the respondents if they are satisfied or not with their current insurance plan (see the Appendix for the exact wording). The relatively small percentage of "don't know" answers to this question (8%) is reassuring and indicates that this variable taps assessments corresponding to the various forms of coverage (Medicare, Medicaid, insurance through employer or union, etc.). As expected, this variable is positively correlated with respondents' evaluations of cares received in the past (tau-b = 0.42, $p < 0.00$) and negatively linked with the expected risk of not getting adequate cares in the future (tau-b = –0.32, $p < 0.00$). It is also strongly correlated with the level of satisfaction with the health care system, as Table 5.1 shows (tau-b = 0.36, $p < 0.00$). Our multivariate model will allow us to disentangle the impact of these variables.

Table 5.1 Satisfaction with the Insurance Plan and Satisfaction with the Health Care System

	Satisfaction with the Health Care System		
Satisfaction with the Insurance Plan	**Very/Fairly Dissatisfied**	**Neither Satisfied nor Dissatisfied**	**Fairly/Very Satisfied**
Very/Fairly dissatisfied/DK	67	18	15
Fairly satisfied	31	23	46
Very satisfied	39	21	41

Notes: Sample sizes are 3,542 in the US. Data are weighted. $\chi 2 = 534.0$ with 4 df; $p < 0.000$ (Cramer's V = 0.29; Kendall's Tau-B = 0.36; $p < 0.000$).

The nature of regional disparities in the levels of satisfaction toward the health care system in the US and Canada is harder to anticipate. Two factors may be at work in this case. The first one is the ideological profile of the four most distinguishable sub-regions of North America: Quebec, the Rest of Canada (ROC), the South, and the Rest of the Union (ROU). According to Grabb and Curtis (2005), Quebec is the most progressive region of North America, the American South is the most conservative, with the other sub-regions, ROC and ROU, being more moderate and more similar. Based on this logic, satisfaction toward the health system is expected to be higher in Quebec and the South because of its government-oriented nature in Canada and its market-based orientation in the US. But as we have seen in Chapter 4, these expectations do not seem to be supported by our data. The lowest level of satisfaction in Canada is to be found in Quebec, while no significant difference in the levels of satisfaction appears in the US between the South and the ROU.

This finding highlights the importance of one important factor that ought to explain the regional disparities in the levels of satisfaction: delivery. In Canada, where the nature of the system is largely consensual, delivery equates performance. The central role of the provinces in the management of the health care system in Canada means that the performance may vary significantly from one region to another. To capture these regional disparities, dummy variables for the major Canadian regions or provinces will be included in the model with the expectation that the level of satisfaction in Quebec should be, all else being equal, lower than in the rest of Canada.

The situation is different in the US. American states have played central and, most importantly, widely varying roles in health care, both in public provision (including the provision of Medicaid and the state children health insurance program) and in regulating private insurance (Jacobs and Callaghan 2013). Briefly stated, since public health provision is relatively similar across Canadian provinces, delivery in this case has a clear valence nature. The provincial governments in Canada are held responsible for the performance (notably wait times) of a system whose basic principles of functioning are consensual. In the US, to the contrary, across-states delivery is positional. There is a clear link, for instance, between party control and the organization of the health care system across American states (though other factors are also at play; see Jacobs and Callaghan 2013), with the health care system in Red states being generally more market-based than in Blue states (see also Aldrich and Coleman Battista 2002; McCarty, Poole, and Rosenthal 2008). This would have called for the inclusion of a "state" variable (49 dummies) in our models. The number of observations in our data is unfortunately too small to make this possible. In order to establish if there is a link between delivery and satisfaction across the states, we have included instead a dummy for the American South. This choice makes sense given the presence in this region of a large number of states who have been reluctant to increase the role of the government in the provision for health care (see Kaiser Family Foundation 2010). If there is a link between market-based delivery and satisfaction toward the health care system, it should manifest itself in a clearer fashion in the South.[1]

Regional disparities can be explored at the individual level, of course. We hypothesize that despite the fact that Americans and Canadians hold roughly similar views about the role of the state in general (see Chapter 4), the divergent orientations taken in the debates about health care in both countries—ideologically-oriented in the US and valence-oriented in Canada—will go a long way toward explaining the marked differences between Americans' and Canadians' opinions regarding their health care system and that of their neighboring country (see Chapters 2 and 4). More specifically, we contend that the framing of the debates on health care, characterized by the central role of partisanship in the US and by varying commitments to equality in access to care in both countries, has left a significant imprint on Americans' and Canadians' views toward their health care system. As a result, because they are basically performance-oriented, we expect that evaluations of past experiences—be they of an egotropic or sociotropic nature—will have a larger impact on Canadians' satisfaction toward their own health care system than for Americans. In the same fashion, given the more intense partisan and ideological polarization in the US regarding the role of the private and public sectors in the health care system, we expect that the effect of individuals' partisan and ideological preferences will have a larger influence on evaluations of the health care system in the US than in Canada.

EXPLAINING SATISFACTION WITH THE HEALTH CARE SYSTEM

In order to test these various theoretical expectations, we develop an empirical model of opinion toward health care. The dependent variable analyzed in this chapter is the respondents' satisfaction toward their own health care system. As was seen in Chapters 1 and 4, Americans and Canadians display different levels of satisfaction toward their health system. To explain these varying levels of satisfaction, we rely on a general model that is constructed based on a series of blocks of explanatory variables, with each block entered one after the other in the analysis. Recall from Chapter 1 that the general form of the multivariate models that will be used, and that will be estimated via ordered logistic regressions, will be the following:

> Opinion (health care) = *f* (SES, egotropic perceptions, general preferences, health care preferences, sociotropic perceptions).

As already explained in Chapter 1, variables are included in the regression analyses according to the logic of block-recursive estimation, based on their "distance" to the dependant variable. The specific form of the models that will now be estimated in this chapter is the following (see the Appendix for a detailed description of the coding of the variables):

> **Satisfaction** = *f* (**SES:** age, gender, race [US only], education, income, public sector employment, region of residence; **Egotropic perceptions:** satisfaction with health insurance plan [US only], assessment of the quality of health care received in the past two years, expectations about the risks of not receiving good health care in the future; **General preferences:** partisan identification, ideological position, role of the state, individualism; **Health care preferences:** health care system, public coverage of health care, symbolism; **Sociotropic perceptions:** evaluation of the quality of care over the past two years).

These successive, block-recursive models have been estimated for respondents in both American and Canadian samples. The models are largely identical for both countries, except for some minor adjustments: ideological identification is measured on a left-right scale in Canada and liberal-conservative scale in the US; a variable for race (black versus others) was included in the US models; regional variables vary from one country to another; a variable measuring satisfaction with the insurance plan has been added in the US; and the "symbolism" variable emphasizes the public character of the health care system in Canada and its private character in the US.

Note, finally, that this general block-recursive model of opinion toward health care will be used again, with appropriate adjustments, in the chapters dealing with evaluation of the neighbor country's health care system (Chapter 6) and with opinion about health care reform in one's own country (Chapter 7).

SATISFACTION WITH HEALTH CARE: MULTIVARIATE FINDINGS

The results of the multivariate models' estimation are presented in Tables 5.2 and 5.3. They are largely in line with the expectations presented in the previous section, including our belief that socioeconomic variables will matter

Table 5.2 Satisfaction with the Canadian Health Care System (Evaluation: Home)

DV: Satisfaction (CAN)	Model 1	Model 2	Model 3	Model 4	Model 5
AB	–0.95***	–0.88***	–0.90***	–0.92***	–0.91***
	(0.12)	(0.14)	(0.14)	(0.14)	(0.14)
BC	–0.51***	–0.44***	–0.42***	–0.43***	–0.50***
	(0.11)	(0.12)	(0.13)	(0.13)	(0.13)
QC	–1.39***	–1.63***	–1.45***	–1.37***	–1.38***
	(0.09)	(0.11)	(0.12)	(0.12)	(0.12)
Atlantic	–0.07	–0.08	–0.03	–0.05	–0.14
	(0.14)	(0.16)	(0.16)	(0.16)	(0.17)
Prairies	–0.15	–0.44**	–0.41*	–0.42*	–0.65***
	(0.15)	(0.17)	(0.17)	(0.17)	(0.18)
Male	0.10	0.02	–0.00	–0.01	–0.01
	(0.07)	(0.08)	(0.08)	(0.08)	(0.08)
Age	0.01**	–0.00	–0.00	–0.00	–0.00
	(0.00)	(0.00)	(0.00)	(0.00)	(0.00)
Education	0.02	–0.01	–0.03	–0.03	–0.01
	(0.02)	(0.02)	(0.02)	(0.02)	(0.03)
Gvt. emp.	0.16	0.02	0.04	0.06	0.04
	(0.11)	(0.12)	(0.12)	(0.12)	(0.12)
Income	0.01	–0.02	–0.02	–0.02	–0.02
	(0.01)	(0.01)	(0.01)	(0.01)	(0.01)
Past2years: egotropic (high)		3.93***	3.90***	3.73***	3.37***
		(0.21)	(0.21)	(0.21)	(0.22)
Risk scale (high)		–3.26***	–3.28***	–3.34***	–2.94***
		(0.18)	(0.18)	(0.18)	(0.19)
CANnopid			–0.38***	–0.35**	–0.31**
			(0.12)	(0.12)	(0.12)
Liberal			0.14	0.06	0.06
			(0.11)	(0.11)	(0.12)
NDP			–0.11	–0.16	0.04
			(0.14)	(0.14)	(0.15)
Bloc			–0.58**	–0.58**	–0.46*
			(0.18)	(0.18)	(0.19)
Green			–0.06	–0.17	–0.21
			(0.40)	(0.40)	(0.42)

DV: Satisfaction (CAN)	Model 1	Model 2	Model 3	Model 4	Model 5
Ideology (right)			–0.18 (0.21)	–0.11 (0.22)	–0.12 (0.22)
Government role (more)			0.08 (0.17)	0.01 (0.17)	0.03 (0.17)
Individualism scale (more)			–0.28 (0.23)	–0.02 (0.24)	–0.04 (0.24)
Gov. insurance plan				–0.05 (0.05)	–0.05 (0.05)
Universal access				0.30 (0.17)	0.32 (0.18)
Public system: symbol				0.14 (0.11)	0.16 (0.12)
Health care system: symbol				0.46*** (0.10)	0.43*** (0.10)
Past2years: sociotropic (high)					2.95*** (0.23)
Cut 1 (constant)	–2.60*** (0.19)	–2.88*** (0.27)	–3.28*** (0.35)	–2.89*** (0.37)	–1.60*** (0.39)
Cut 2 (constant)	–1.17*** (0.18)	–1.06*** (0.26)	–1.44*** (0.34)	–1.04** (0.37)	0.33 (0.39)
Cut 3 (constant)	–0.26 (0.17)	0.00 (0.26)	–0.37 (0.34)	0.05 (0.37)	1.46*** (0.39)
Cut 4 (constant)	2.18*** (0.18)	3.15*** (0.26)	2.84*** (0.34)	3.27*** (0.37)	4.82*** (0.40)
N	2,881	2,449	2,449	2,449	2,406
Pseudo R^2	0.10	0.41	0.42	0.43	0.47

Notes: Data are weighted. Entries are ordered logistic regression coefficients with standard errors in parentheses. Pseudo R^2 are Nagelkerke. *p < 0.05, **p < 0.01, ***p < 0.001. For the description of the variables, see the Appendix.

more in the US whereas regional variables will matter more in Canada (see column 1 of Tables 5.2 and 5.3). In the US, no significant regional divide is apparent but several socioeconomic cleavages (gender, race, and especially income) show up as being statistically significant or closed to. The fact that age in Canada and in the US, each contribute to increase the level

Table 5.3 Satisfaction with the American Health Care System (Evaluation: Home)

DV: Satisfaction (US)	Model 1	Model 2	Model 3	Model 4	Model 5
South	–0.05 (0.07)	–0.03 (0.08)	–0.07 (0.08)	–0.05 (0.08)	–0.08 (0.08)
Male	0.23*** (0.06)	0.19 (0.07)	0.19* (0.08)	0.15* (0.08)	0.07 (0.08)
Age	0.01* (0.00)	–0.01** (0.00)	–0.01** (0.00)	–0.01** (0.00)	–0.00 (0.00)
Education	–0.03 (0.02)	–0.05 (0.03)	–0.02 (0.03)	–0.02 (0.03)	–0.03 (0.03)
Black	0.22* (0.10)	0.41*** (0.11)	0.54*** (0.12)	0.46*** (0.12)	0.39** (0.13)
Gvt. emp.	0.18 (0.14)	–0.25 (0.16)	–0.27 (0.16)	–0.19 (0.16)	–0.19 (0.17)
Income	0.05*** (0.01)	–0.01 (0.01)	0.02 (0.02)	0.02 (0.01)	–0.01 (0.01)
SatINS		1.84*** (0.13)	1.71*** (0.13)	1.64*** (0.13)	1.53*** (0.14)
Past2years: quality (high)		1.92*** (0.21)	1.84*** (0.21)	1.77*** (0.21)	1.22*** (0.22)
Risk scale (high)		–1.68*** (0.14)	–1.61*** (0.15)	–1.74*** (0.15)	–1.42*** (0.15)
USAnopid			–0.10 (0.10)	0.00 (0.10)	–0.04 (0.10)
Democrat			0.23* (0.12)	0.28* (0.12)	0.20 (0.12)
Ideology (conservative)			0.54*** (0.17)	0.24 (0.17)	0.30 (0.18)
Government role (more)			–0.07 (0.15)	0.06 (0.16)	0.02 (0.17)
Individualism scale (more)			1.21*** (0.20)	0.88*** (0.21)	0.79*** (0.21)
Gov. insurance plan				–0.04 (0.04)	–0.05 (0.05)
Universal access				–0.46** (0.16)	–0.44** (0.16)

DV: Satisfaction (US)	**Model 1**	**Model 2**	**Model 3**	**Model 4**	**Model 5**
Private system: symbol				0.53***	0.47***
				(0.08)	(0.09)
Health care system: symbol				0.41***	0.28***
				(0.09)	(0.09)
Past2years: sociotropic (high)					2.68***
					(0.20)
Cut 1 (constant)	–1.20***	–1.22***	–0.47	–1.00**	–0.14
	(0.17)	(0.25)	(0.32)	(0.34)	(0.35)
Cut 2 (constant)	0.08	0.39	1.17***	0.78*	1.63***
	(0.16)	(0.25)	(0.32)	(0.34)	(0.35)
Cut 3 (constant)	1.00***	1.35***	2.16***	1.79***	2.67***
	(0.16)	(0.25)	(0.32)	(0.34)	(0.35)
Cut 4 (constant)	3.00***	3.72***	4.57***	4.26***	5.25***
	(0.17)	(0.26)	(0.33)	(0.35)	(0.37)
N	3,265	2,507	2,507	2,507	2,466
Pseudo R^2	0.02	0.30	0.32	0.34	0.39

Notes: Data are weighted. Entries are ordered logistic regression coefficients with standard errors in parentheses. Pseudo R^2 are Nagelkerke. *$p < 0.05$, **$p < 0.01$, ***$p < 0.001$. For the description of the variables, see the Appendix.

of satisfaction toward the health care system is interesting as it may signal that senior Americans and Canadians express positive feelings toward the universal coverage they benefit from in both countries (thanks to Medicare in the US and the public system in Canada).

We have posited in the previous section that evaluations of the health care systems will be more performance-oriented in Canada and more delivery-oriented in the US. Accordingly, we expect that citizens' personal experience with the system will be more strongly tied to evaluations of the health care system in Canada than in the US. The results for the impact of egotropic perceptions confirm this hypothesis (see Tables 5.2 and 5.3, column 2). The coefficients for both retrospective (Past 2 years) and prospective (Risk scale) egotropic perceptions are strong and significant in both countries, but their impact is clearly larger in Canada (coefficients of 3.93 and –3.26) than in the US (coefficients of 1.92 and –1.68).

A reasonable assumption would be that this difference is due to the inclusion of a powerful, additional variable in the US model, namely the one measuring respondents' satisfaction toward their health insurance coverage (SatINS). It is true that this variable exerts a major impact on respondents' satisfaction toward the health care system in the US. As can be seen in Table 5.3, the magnitude of its coefficient (1.84) is virtually similar to retrospective and prospective perceptions. The exclusion of the "insurance" variable, though, does not alter the conclusion about the larger impact of egotropic perceptions in Canada. The coefficients for both variables increase significantly, standing at 2.81 and –2.20, but are still clearly lower than for Canada. Furthermore, the increase in the pseudo R^2 when this second block of variables is added to the model is still higher in Canada (0.31) than in the US (0.28) even with the inclusion of the "insurance" variable. The results thus neatly show that both Americans and Canadians rely heavily on their personal experience to form global judgments about the performance of their health care system. But the link between their personal situation and these assessments is slightly stronger in Canada. And the results also neatly show the crucial importance of medical insurance, either public or private, as a determinant of individuals' satisfaction toward the health care system in the US.

We can also see that opinions about health care seem to be more structured by political attitudes in the US than in Canada. Ideology and individualism are strongly tied to evaluations of the health care system in the US, but not at all in Canada (see column 3 of Tables 5.2 and 5.3). The strength of the relationship between individualism and opinions about the health care system is particularly striking in the US (coefficient of 1.21). These results provide evidence that opinions on health care are more ideologically polarized in the US, in the sense that basic political attitudes are more strongly related to Americans' overall satisfaction with the way health care is run in their country than is the case in Canada.

The traces of partisan and ideological polarization on views of the health care systems are also apparent when variables directly tied to attitudes toward the role of public and private sectors in the functioning of the health system are introduced in the estimation (see column 4 of Tables 5.2 and 5.3). The variable "government insurance plan," which precisely gets at the respective roles of the public and private sectors in health care, is tied to satisfaction toward the health care system in the US (significant coefficient of –0.12), but not in Canada. Similarly, a variable measuring respondents' level of agreement with the notion that the government should act to ensure that health care is universally available is significant in the US (despite the presence of numerous controls), but not in Canada. Thus, preferences regarding the role of the public and private sectors in health care more strongly color opinions about health care in the US.

Another revealing finding is the fact that the only variable in this fourth block that has a significant impact on satisfaction toward the health care system in Canada is the one that measures agreement with the idea that the health care system is a symbol of Canadian unity. Interestingly, the same item is also significant for the US, with that variable being based on a question stating that "market-based health care is part of what it means to be American and reflects our core values." The results are neat. The four variables within the block measuring specific attitudes about the workings of the health care system are significant for the US and contribute collectively to an increase of 0.03 to the pseudo R^2, whereas the single variable that is found to be significant for the Canadian sample barely contributes to increase the proportion of explained variance.

The results presented here seem to confirm that health care has the characteristics of a valence issue in Canada and a positional issue in the US. If this characterization is correct, then the effect of sociotropic perceptions—the respondents' assessment of the quality of health care in the past two years—should be greater in Canada than in US. The results indicate that the impact of this variable is almost the same in both countries, though a bit higher in Canada (2.95 versus 2.68; see column 5 in Tables 5.2 and 5.3). This finding is perhaps not surprising given the proximity between this variable and the dependent variable. Still, the inclusion of sociotropic perceptions in the model is useful to establish our findings about the determinants of individual opinions about health care on a strong footing for the next two chapters.

So far we have presented regression coefficients and pseudo R^2 values to indicate the impact of different types of variables on individuals' assessment of the performance of their health care system. A more intuitive measure is the change in the probability that a typical respondent will express his satisfaction toward the health care system when the value of a given explanatory variable changes from its minimal to its maximal value. In the case of a simple dichotomous variable, gender for example, a variation from its minimal to its maximal value means being a male (gender equals 1) instead of a female (gender equals 0). In this case, the change in probability reflects the lower or higher level of satisfaction, all else being equal, of males compared to females about the performance of the health care system.

These changes in probabilities are displayed in Tables 5.4 and 5.5. Given that the dependent variable is ordinal—it is formed of five categories going from the highest level of dissatisfaction (value of 0) to the highest level of satisfaction (value of 1) toward the health care system—the interpretation of these coefficients represents the change in the probability that a respondent will express the highest level of satisfaction with the health care system when the value of an explanatory variable changes from its minimal to its maximal value. For the egotropic retrospective variable (Past2years) for instance, the values in column 2 of Tables 5.4 and 5.5 mean that the probability that a typical Canadian or an American respondent expresses the highest level of satisfaction about the health care system (very satisfied) increases, all else being equal, by thirty-four percentage points in Canada and fourteen points in the US when his evaluation of the quality of the care he has received in the past two years moves from very poor to excellent. This result is interesting on three accounts. First, it shows that transforming the regression coefficients into changes in probabilities do not alter any of the substantive conclusions discussed so far. Second, it reiterates the point that past experiences with the health care system looms large in a citizen's evaluation of

Table 5.4 Change in Probabilities Related to Satisfaction with the Canadian Health Care System (Evaluation: Home)

DV: Satisfaction (CAN)	Model 1	Model 2	Model 3	Model 4	Model 5
AB	–0.09	–0.08	–0.08	–0.08	–0.07
BC	–0.05	–0.04	–0.04	–0.04	–0.04
QC	–0.14	–0.14	–0.12	–0.12	–0.11
Atlantic	–0.01	–0.01	–0.00	–0.00	–0.01
Prairies	–0.01	–0.04	–0.04	–0.04	–0.05
Male	0.01	0.00	–0.00	–0.00	–0.00
Age	0.001	–0.000	–0.000	–0.002	–0.000
Education	0.00	–0.00	–0.00	–0.00	–0.00
Gvt. emp.	0.02	0.00	0.00	0.01	0.00
Income	0.001	–0.002	–0.002	–0.002	–0.002
Past2years: quality (high)		0.34	0.33	0.32	0.27
Risk scale (high)		–0.28	–0.28	–0.28	–0.24
CANnopid			–0.03	–0.03	–0.03
Liberal			0.01	0.01	0.00
NDP			–0.01	–0.01	0.00
Bloc			–0.05	–0.05	–0.04
Green			–0.01	–0.01	–0.02
Ideology (right)			–0.02	–0.01	–0.01
Government role (more)			0.01	0.00	0.00
Individualism scale (more)			–0.02	–0.00	–0.00
Gov. insurance plan				–0.00	–0.00
Universal access				0.03	0.03
Public system: symbol				0.01	0.01
Health care system: symbol				0.04	0.03
Past2years: sociotropic (high)					0.24

Notes: Entries in the table are the changes in probability that the dependent variable takes its highest value (very satisfied) when an explanatory variable varies from its minimum to its maximum value. All calculations were performed with Stata 11.0.

its overall performance. Third, it demonstrates once again that Canadians' assessments of their health care system are more performance-oriented than in the US. The results also show the important influence of insurance health coverage on the level of satisfaction toward the health care system in the US.

Table 5.5 Change in Probabilities Related to Satisfaction with the American Health Care System (Evaluation: Home)

DV: Satisfaction (US)	Model 1	Model 2	Model 3	Model 4	Model 5
South	–0.00	–0.00	–0.00	–0.00	–0.01
Male	0.02	0.01	0.01	0.01	0.00
Age	0.000	–0.000	–0.001	–0.001	–0.000
Education	–0.00	–0.00	–0.00	–0.00	–0.00
Black	0.02	0.03	0.04	0.03	0.03
Gvt. emp.	0.01	–0.02	–0.02	–0.01	–0.01
Income	0.003	0.001	0.001	–0.001	–0.001
SatINS		0.13	0.12	0.12	0.10
Past2years: quality (high)		0.14	0.13	0.12	0.08
Risk scale (high)		–0.12	–0.12	–0.12	–0.10
USAnopid			–0.01	0.00	–0.00
Democrat			0.02	0.02	0.01
Ideology (conservative)			0.04	0.02	0.02
Government role (more)			–0.01	0.00	0.00
Individualism scale (more)			0.09	0.06	0.05
Gov. insurance plan				–0.00	–0.00
Universal access				–0.03	–0.03
Private system: symbol				0.04	0.03
Health care system: symbol				0.03	0.02
Past2years: sociotropic (high)					0.18

Notes: Entries in the table are the changes in probability that the dependent variable takes its highest value (very satisfied) when an explanatory variable varies from its minimum to its maximum value. All calculations were performed with Stata 11.0.

The values in column 2 of Table 5.5 show that the impact of this variable (0.13) is as strong as the evaluation of the quality of health care received in the past (0.14) and expected for the future (–0.12). This result helps to understand why the questions of insurance and coverage are central in the debate about health care reform in the US.

Overall, results in Tables 5.4 and 5.5 confirm our observations based on the regression coefficients. Satisfaction toward the health care system varies more among regions in Canada and across social groups in the US, and its assessment seems more performance-based in Canada (the changes in probability for the retrospective egotropic and sociotropic perceptions are 0.27, –0.24 and 0.24, and 0.08, –0.10 and 0.18 in Canada and the US, respectively; see column 5 in Tables 5.4 and 5.5).

The results of models exploring the sources of satisfaction toward the American and Canadian health care systems thus largely conform to our general expectations. The more polarized ideological and partisan environment in the US with regard to the role of the public and private sector in health care, combined with the priming effect of partisan messages in the flurry of debates led by President Obama, can explain both the large role that ideological outlooks play in structuring public opinion on this issue and the fact that the issue of health care has more characteristics of a positional issue in the US than in Canada.

CONCLUSION

This chapter has tried to bridge a gap in the literature by offering a general model that can explain Americans' and Canadians' satisfaction with the way health care is run in their own country. This model brings together variables that refer to socioeconomic status, ideological and partisan preferences, and personal experience with the health care system. The results point to two general conclusions. The first conclusion concerns respondents' high level of sophistication in their evaluations of health care–related issues. The findings related to the multifaceted nature of these evaluations—egotropic, sociotropic, retrospective, and prospective—clearly suggest that more attention needs to be paid to the way in which citizens position themselves with regard to this question, not only because of its importance but also in order to better understand how individuals form opinions on different issues.

Another conclusion of this chapter has to do with the link between the political context and opinions on a given issue. Americans' and Canadians' expectations regarding the performance criteria of health care systems seem to overlap to a great deal. However, they are expressed in two different contexts: one where the constituent principles of the health care system are based on consensus and the other where they separate rather distinct ideological and partisan groups. The more structured character of Americans' opinions on health care seems to result from this polarization, which the recent debate over health care reform has certainly accentuated even more.

The results in this chapter highlight again the divergent role of partisanship in the formation of health care attitudes in Canada and the US, almost negligible in the first case, central in the second. They also signal the varying commitments to equality in access to care across both countries. In Canada, coverage is universal. In the US, it varies according to the nature of an individual's health insurance scheme. It is not surprising, then, that health insurance and coverage are central to any collective deliberation about health care in the US, while these questions are much less important in Canada. However, in spite of these differences, one fact remains constant. Overall, Americans are less satisfied with their health care system than Canadians are and, as we shall see in the remainder of this book, they are more inclined to want a large-scale reform.

NOTE

1. We have also tested the possibility that differences emerge among other regions—Northeast, Midwest, East—but none of these variables even approached statistical significance. This result might be partly due to across-states variations among these broad regions and calls for detailed state-by-state analyses of health care delivery and satisfaction toward the health care system in the US (see Jacobs and Callaghan 2013). It could also be due to the "nationalization" of the health care debate in the US in the last few years. It may be the case that this debate has "primed" national considerations over local realities for many Americans over the last few years.

6 Americans' and Canadians' Views of the Other's Health Care System

Past chapters have made clear the differences in Americans' and Canadians' attitudes about their own health care system. Our work thus far has been able to build on a small but valuable literature on health care attitudes in the United States and Canada. We now shift gears, however, and focus on a subject that has rarely, if ever, found its way into analysis of public attitudes on health care. We focus here not on Americans' and Canadians' attitudes about their own health care system but on their attitudes about each other's health care system.

A comparison of Americans' and Canadians' opinions on the health care system of their neighbor is particularly interesting because it is a very rare case of citizens in one country having a relatively well-defined opinion regarding a specific public policy of another country. And, importantly, these outward-looking attitudes matter to the development of health care policy, particularly in the US.

These considerations add to our interest in studying these crossed signals. It will also allow us to examine, in Chapter 7, a hypothesis never before tested, touching on the possible influence of respondents' perceptions of their neighboring country's health care system on the relevance of reforming their own system (or not). All other things equal, is it possible that Americans who have a positive image of the Canadian health care system would be more inclined to reform their own? This speculation clearly adds to the interest of studying cross-border perceptions about the health care systems in Canada and the US.

The present chapter is divided into three parts. First, despite the scarcity of the literature, we will try to identify the factors susceptible of moving cross-border opinion on health care in North America. Second, we will examine the opinions of Americans about the Canadian health care system, and vice versa, in a descriptive fashion. Finally, we will explore the determinants of these perceptions with a carefully designed multivariate model that is in line with the one just developed in our previous chapter.

WHAT MOVES CROSS-BORDER OPINION?

A first factor at play in explaining cross-border perceptions has to do with the availability of information about the health care system of the neighboring country in both Canada and the US, as well as the level of citizen attentiveness in both countries toward this information. Given the relative sizes of Canada and the US and the prominent role of the US in today's world, one may expect that Canadians will be on average more knowledgeable about their southern neighbor than Americans will be about Canada. The more widespread diffusion of information on the American health care system in Canada, notably in the context of debate over its reform (Marmor 1993), should reinforce this asymmetry. In brief, we should expect Canadians to be more opinionated about the US's health care system than Americans would be about the Canadian system.

A second expectation has to do with the relative importance of personal experience and partisan and ideological preferences in the formation of cross-border perceptions. Schlesinger and Lee (1993) found that individuals' opinions about health care depend on the nature of their experiences with the health care system itself (see also Chapter 3), alongside their political and partisan preferences. Given their "unobtrusive" character (Zucker 1978), perceptions of Canadians and Americans about the health care system in their neighboring country are expected to be more influenced by individuals' partisan and ideological preferences than by evaluations of actual health care provision in their own country. In other words, personal experience, a key factor in explaining satisfaction toward one's own health care as we have seen previously, is not expected to play an important role as a judgmental shortcut that helps citizens to form opinions about the situation of health care abroad. These perceptions are expected to be driven largely, but not exclusively, by projections based on political preferences.

Given what we have seen in preceding chapters, this pattern is expected to be more pronounced in the US. Higher ideological polarization in the US regarding public policies in general (Bartels 2008) and the functioning of the health care system in particular (Jacobs and Shapiro 2000; see also preceding chapters) are expected to leave an especially visible imprint on Americans' perceptions of the Canadian health care system. Moreover, the fact that this polarization has been "primed" by the recent debate over the health care reform proposed by Barack Obama should make an even larger difference with regard to the impact of political preferences on cross-border perceptions in the US when compared to Canada.

The fact that cross-border perceptions are largely derived from political preferences does not mean that they are entirely "artificial." There are good reasons to believe that Americans' and Canadians' perceptions of the health care system of their neighboring country are "genuine." Previous studies (Marmor 1993; Angus Reid 2009) have shown that most Americans, either liberal or conservative, tend to be aware of the collective orientation of the Canadian system and share views about its merits (e.g., universal coverage) and limits (e.g., waiting time). Most Canadians see the American health care system as individualistic and market based, efficient for those who are adequately covered, but unfair for many.

Because of the distinct nature of the American and Canadian health care systems, the impact of most variables on cross-border perceptions should vary from one country to another. The US system is predominantly market based and characterized by larger disparities in terms of accessibility, whereas the Canadian system is more collective and explicitly devised to guarantee universal coverage. Consequently, the variables usually linked to more rightist orientations (such as age, income, individualism, negative attitudes toward the state, etc.) will be negatively related to favorable opinions toward the Canadian health care system among Americans and positively related to positive opinions toward the American health care system in Canada. In other words, richer Canadians are expected to be favorably disposed toward the American health care system, with the opposite being true for more affluent Americans.

AMERICANS' AND CANADIANS' VIEWS ON HEALTH CARE SYSTEMS IN NORTH AMERICA

Americans' and Canadians' opinions toward each other's health care system have not been the subject of much systematic study. That said, in spite of its limits, a study from Angus Reid sheds some interesting light on this issue. In their study, respondents in both countries are asked first to express their general opinion on their own health care system and that of their neighboring country. They are then asked to determine in which country they would be better placed to receive the best treatment without much delay (Angus Reid 2009). The results show that Canadians have a better opinion of their own health care system than Americans do. They also show that Canadians have a largely negative opinion about the health care system in the US, while Americans seem to have a much more positive perception of the Canadian health care system. Finally, the Angus Reid data show that the main advantage of the Canadian health care system for respondents in both countries was its accessibility to care, while the main strength of the American system for respondents in both countries seems to be fewer delays in receiving treatment. (Note that these findings are perfectly in line with what we have seen in our own data thus far.)

The data from our study allow for a somewhat more detailed examination of these perceptions. The data presented in Table 6.1 show respondents' overall impression of their neighboring country's health care system, gauged with the help of the following question: "What is your overall impression of the health care system in Canada (United States)?

Table 6.1 Opinions about Health Care in Canada and the US (%)

	Canadian Sample		American Sample	
	Canadian HCS	American HCS	American HCS	Canadian HCS
Very positive	20	2	6	15
Moderately positive	61	12	34	32
Moderately negative	14	40	37	13
Very negative	3	33	19	8
Don't know	2	13	4	33

Notes: Sample sizes are 3,522 and 3,542 for Canada and the US, respectively. Data are weighted. Question Wording: What is your overall impression of the health care system in [Canada/USA]?

Very positive, moderately positive, moderately negative, or very negative?" In order to have a base of comparison to put things into perspective, the same question was also used to measure respondents' opinions toward their own health care system.

The results of Table 6.1 are interesting in several ways. First, they confirm, as we have seen, that Canadians have a more favorable opinion of their own health care system than the Americans do of theirs. While more than eight Canadians out of ten (81%) expressed a positive opinion of their own health care system, only four Americans out of ten (40%) did the same for their own system. A second finding has to do with respondents' inclination to express an opinion on their own health care system. The rate of non-response is barely 2% in Canada and 4% in the US. The propensity of respondents to express an opinion about the health care system of their neighboring country is evidently less obvious. As expected, Canadians expressed an opinion on the American health care system more often than Americans did with regard to the Canadian health care system. The rate of non-response is 13% in Canada, while it reached 33% in the US.

The results showing respondents' opinions of the health care system of their neighboring country are telling. The contrast is striking between Canadians' massively negative opinion of the American health care system and Americans' mostly positive opinion of the Canadian health care system. There are five times more Canadians who have a negative opinion of the American health care system than those who have the opposite opinion (73% versus 14%), while there are twice as many Americans who have a favorable opinion of the Canadian system than those who have the opposite opinion (47% versus 21%).

What factors can explain such a large divergence of opinion between respondents in both countries? Several explanations can be examined

Table 6.2 Opinions about the Main Advantage of the Canadian and the American Health Care Systems (%)

	Canadian Sample		American Sample	
	Canadian HCS	American HCS	American HCS	Canadian HCS
Quicker access	3	43	17	2
Higher quality	6	11	23	6
Possibility to choose	4	10	17	3
More affordable	77	7	5	51
No advantage	3	15	14	13
Don't know	7	14	24	25

Notes: Sample sizes are 3,522 and 3,542 for Canada and the US, respectively. Data are weighted. Question Wording: In your opinion, what is the main advantage of the [Canadian/American] health care system compared to the [Canadian/American] one? Quicker access to a trained specialist, higher quality health care, possibility of choosing your doctor or your hospital, more affordable healthcare, no advantage.

descriptively before turning to multivariate analysis. The results presented in Table 6.2 provide a few possibilities. The data in this table show the responses given to two questions that ask survey participants in both countries to name the main advantage of their own health care system, followed by that of their neighboring country. They were given the following choices: (1) quicker access to health care, (2) higher quality of health care, (3) possibility to choose your physician or hospital, and (4) more affordable care.

Two things stand out from the responses received. The first has to do with the sheer number of respondents who were incapable of identifying an advantage of their own health care system when compared to that of their neighboring country. This percentage is almost four times larger in the US (38%) than it is in Canada (barely 10%). This result is significant because it speaks volumes not about the health care system of the neighboring country, but about that of the respondent's home country. The inability of a large number of Americans to identify even one advantage of their own system is particularly revealing.

The results having to do with identifying the main advantage of American and Canadian health care systems are no less enlightening. The convergence of respondents' views in both countries about the Canadian health care system is particularly clear. Almost eight Canadians out of ten (77%) are of the opinion that the Canadian health care system's strength lies in its affordability; this opinion is also widely held in the US, where a majority of respondents (51%) agree. This convergence is also more remarkable if one compares the most attentive publics in both countries by excluding non-respondents (7% in Canada and 25% in the US). In this case, 82% of Canadian respondents and 68% of American respondents who have an opinion on the Canadian health care system identify its affordability as its main advantage.

According to the results, the American health care system does not seem to have as clear of an advantage, at least in the eyes of Americans. Almost one American in four (24%) could not identify an advantage. The distribution in the responses of those who did name an advantage is not any less revealing. A reasonably equal number of respondents opted for its quality of care (24%), quicker access to care (17%), and the possibility to choose one's own doctor (17%) as the American health care system's main advantage. Canadians' views of the American health care system are clearer; a strong plurality of respondents (43%), which reaches 49% among those who actually expressed an opinion, stated that quicker access to health care is a distinct advantage of the American health care system when compared to that of their own country.

The data in Tables 6.1 and 6.2 provide some interesting findings about cross-border perceptions of North American health care systems. First, it is clear that Canadians seem to know more about the American health care system than Americans do about the Canadian one. It is also clear that the Canadian system has a distinct advantage over the American system, which is the affordability of its care. Furthermore, a significant number of Canadians believe that quicker access to health care is the main advantage of the American health care system. These findings seem to suggest that respondents place greater weight on cost rather than wait times in their evaluation of health care systems. This hierarchy of evaluation criteria could explain Americans' largely positive view of the Canadian health care system and Canadians' considerable reluctance toward that of the US.

The data presented in Table 6.3 seem to support this interpretation. The first part shows the responses to a question asking respondents if the American health care system is overall better, worse, or practically the same as the Canadian health care system. The view of Canadians is remarkably clear. Seven times more Canadians believe that their health care system is superior (72% versus 7%). Americans' evaluations are more divided, but also favor the Canadian system; about four Americans out of ten (39%) think that the Canadian system is better versus one respondent in four (25%) who thinks the opposite.

The data in the second part of the table add an explanatory element to these evaluations. The advantage of the Canadian system, from both sides of the border, stands out when the comparison has to do with equality rather than efficiency of health care systems. In this case, Canadians' opinions become absolute, since twenty times more Canadians think that their health care system is more equitable than that of the US (85% versus 4%). However, the results from the US, less spectacular, show just how

Table 6.3 Evaluations of the Canadian and the American Health Care Systems (%)

Panel A. Best System
For you personally, do you think that the American health care system is better, worse or much the same as the Canadian health care system?

	Canadian Sample	American Sample
Better	7	25
Same	10	11
Worse	72	39
Don't know	10	25

Panel B. Efficiency and Fairness
Overall, in your view, which health care system is the most effective [the fairest], the Canadian or the American?

	Canadian sample		American sample	
	Most Effective	Fairest	Most Effective	Fairest
Canadian	77	85	37	40
American	9	4	31	2
Don't know	15	11	32	34

Notes: Sample sizes are 3,522 and 3,542 for Canada and the US, respectively. Data are weighted.

clearly framing the issue in terms of equality brings out more positive opinions about the Canadian system than framing it in terms of efficiency would.

The opinions examined until now have reflected the overall impressions of the survey respondents. What about respondents' evaluations of more specific aspects of the health care system in their neighboring country? The data in Table 6.4 offer a first look at this information. This table shows the responses to a series of questions asking respondents if the proportion of citizens worried about paying for health care, being covered by health insurance (either private or public) when in need, having access to high-quality care and appropriate medication, and being treated quickly is larger, smaller, or the same in their own country when compared to their neighboring country. The results are clear. Canadians largely believe that there are more people concerned with the cost and quality of health care in the US than in their own country, with the only downside to the Canadian system being long wait times. Remarkably, this assessment is also shared by Americans, who believe that their fellow citizens are more concerned with a series of questions related to health care (cost, coverage, access to

Table 6.4 Perceptions of Canadians' and Americans' Problems with Their Health Care Systems (%)

Panel A. Canadian Sample

From what you know, would you say that the Canadian population that is worried about [being able to pay for their medical care][the coverage of their health care needs] is higher, lower or about the same as in the United States?

From what you know, would you say that the proportion of the population unable [to afford the care it needs][to receive the most effective drugs][to receive high quality health care][to wait longer than reasonable to get health care services] in Canada is higher, lower or about the same as in the United States?

	Pay	*Coverage*	*Afford*	*Drugs*	*Quality*	*Wait*
Higher	8	9	6	8	11	41
Same	14	15	13	19	16	20
Lower	70	69	73	62	63	24
Don't know	8	8	8	12	10	15

Panel B. American Sample

From what you know, would you say that the American population that is worried about [being able to pay for their medical care][the coverage of their health care needs] is higher, lower or about the same as in the United States?

From what you know, would you say that the proportion of the population unable [to afford the care it needs][to receive the most effective drugs][to receive high quality health care][to wait longer than reasonable to get health care services] in the United States is higher, lower or about the same as in the Canada?

	Pay	*Coverage*	*Afford*	*Drugs*	*Quality*	*Wait*
Higher	62	59	46	44	40	22
Same	12	13	18	16	17	18
Lower	10	11	7	12	17	33
Don't know	16	16	28	29	27	27

Notes: Sample sizes are 3,522 and 3,542 for Canada and the US, respectively. Data are weighted.

quality medication and care) than Canadian citizens are. The only exception is with regard to wait times, which are shorter in the US. Once again, it seems clear that the Canadian health care system's superiority emerges when respondents are asked to evaluate the system sociotropically rather than egotropically.

The data in Table 6.5 cast some light on this interesting point. Survey respondents' evaluations of their neighboring country's health care system were measured in two different ways. The first way consisted of asking

Table 6.5 Perceptions of Canadians' and Americans' Opinions about the Best Health Care System (%)

Panel A. Canadian Sample (Egotropic Perceptions)

Suppose you or a member of your family become sick today. From what you know, which health care system would be better at dealing with the following problems, the Canadian or the American? [offering you affordable health care][making available the most effective drugs][offering you high quality health care][allowing you quick access to a trained specialist][allowing you to choose your doctor or your hospital][providing you a comprehensive, guaranteed and affordable insurance covering your health care needs].

	Affordable Care	*Effective Drugs*	*Quality Care*	*Quick Access*		*More Choice*	*Compre-hensive Insurance*	*Average*
				Specialist	*Surgery*			
Canadian	89	55	53	32	33	44	77	55
American	2	23	27	50	50	35	5	27
Don't know	9	23	20	18	18	21	18	18

Panel B. American Sample (Egotropic Perceptions)

Suppose you or a member of your family become sick today. From what you know, which health care system would be better at dealing with the following problems, the Canadian or the American? [offering you affordable health care][making available the most effective drugs][offering you high quality health care][allowing you quick access to a trained specialist][allowing you to choose your doctor or your hospital][providing you a comprehensive, guaranteed and affordable insurance covering your health care needs].

	Affordable Care	*Effective Drugs*	*Quality Care*	*Quick Access*		*More Choice*	*Compre-hensive Insurance*	*Average*
				Specialist	*Surgery*			
Canadian	49	31	20	18	19	17	42	27
American	23	38	49	52	51	53	27	41
Don't know	28	30	30	30	30	30	31	32

Panel C. Canadian Sample (Sociotropic Perceptions)

Now, not thinking about yourself and your family but about the population in general. From what you know, which health care system would be better at dealing with the following problems for everybody (rich and poor), the Canadian or the American? [offering you affordable health care][making available the most effective drugs][offering you high quality health care][allowing you quick access to a trained specialist][allowing you to choose your doctor or your hospital][providing you a comprehensive, guaranteed and affordable insurance covering your health care needs].

	Affordable Care	*Effective Drugs*	*Quality Care*	*Quick Access*		*More Choice*	*Compre-hensive Insurance*	*Average*
				Specialist	*Surgery*			
Canadian	87	64	73	49	51	51	78	65
American	2	17	11	33	32	28	5	18
Don't know	11	20	16	18	18	21	17	17

Panel D. American Sample (Sociotropic Perceptions)

Now, not thinking about yourself and your family but about the population in general. From what you know, which health care system would be better at dealing with the following problems for everybody (rich and poor), the Canadian or the American? [offering you affordable health care][making available the most effective drugs][offering you high quality health care][allowing you quick access to a trained specialist][allowing you to choose your doctor or your hospital] [providing you a comprehensive, guaranteed and affordable insurance covering your health care needs].

	Affordable Care	*Effective Drugs*	*Quality Care*	*Quick Access*		*More Choice*	*Compre-hensive Insurance*	*Average*
				Specialist	*Surgery*			
Canadian	53	36	35	23	25	21	48	34
American	18	32	34	44	43	46	21	35
Don't know	29	32	31	33	32	33	32	31

Notes: Sample sizes are 3,522 and 3,542 for Canada and the US, respectively. Data are weighted.

respondents which of the two systems offered the most advantageous situation for them should they or a member of their family become sick. Questions were then meant to lead respondents to determine which of the two systems would allow them or a member of their family to obtain the most affordable care, be prescribed the most effective medication, benefit from high-quality care, have quick access to a specialist or a surgery, be able to choose their own doctor or hospital, and overall benefit from a health care system that offers affordable care with adequate coverage. The second version used the same categories, but asked respondents which of the two systems would offer the most advantage to not just themselves or their family but all of their country's citizens, rich or poor.

The data in Table 6.5 not only confirm but also nuance the results shown in previous tables. These data show that Canadians overwhelmingly believe that their health care system allows them to be cared for at a lower cost than in the US (89% versus 2%), while a strong plurality of them also believe that it also assures them better access to medication (55% versus 23%) and to quality care (53% to 27%; see Part A of the table). Canadians are more divided over which system gives them the widest choice of doctor or hospital; 44% of them believe that the Canadian system best assures this freedom of choice, while 35% believe that the American system is in a better position to do so. Shorter wait times to see a specialist or to have a surgical procedure is a distinct advantage of the American system: half of Canadians surveyed (50%) believe that one could see a specialist or have a surgery faster in the US than in Canada, while almost one respondent in three (32% and 33% respectively) believed the opposite. Finally, Canadians largely believe (77% versus 5%) in the superiority of their system assuring them the best access to health care at the lowest cost.

At first glance, the portrait that emerges from the responses of the American survey respondents (Table 6.5, Part B) seems more nuanced than one might be led to believe. To them, the Canadian health care system's affordability is the main attribute that distinguishes it from the American system. Around half of the respondents believe that they would receive care at a lower cost in Canada (49%), while a little less than a quarter (23%) believe the opposite. American respondents see their own system to be superior to the Canadian one, in all other aspects such as access to medication and quality care (38% and 49% versus 31% and 20%), quick access to a specialist or a surgery (52% and 51% versus 18% and 19%), and a better chance of choosing one's own doctor or hospital (53% versus 17%). However, the advantage of the Canadian system reappears when American respondents are asked to identify the system that would give them "a comprehensive, guaranteed and affordable insurance plan covering their health care needs." More than four Americans in ten (42%) believe that the Canadian health care system best meets these requirements, while slightly more than one quarter (27%) would opt for their own health care system (31% of the respondents did not make a choice or said they were unable to decide).

The figures in the first two parts of Table 6.5 lead one to believe that Americans' and Canadians' opinions on the relative merits of health care in the US and Canada are perhaps not as divided as the preceding results would make them out to be. However, other results in this table (Parts C and D) confirm our previous findings. The advantages of the Canadian health care system over that of the US are clearly seen once again when the question emphasizes the entire population and not the individual and their family.

The Canadian data are telling. With the exception of the question of cost, where there is a ceiling effect, Canadians' opinions of their own health care system become more favorable when looked at from a sociotropic, rather than egotropic, perspective. In this case, the Canadian system seems to be the more favored system with regard to all the criteria examined. The percentage of respondents who opted for the Canadian system rises on average ten percentage points (from 55% to 65%), with the largest gains being in access to quality care (+20) and wait times to see a specialist or have a surgical procedure (+17 and +18); this is where we can see a reversal of the American system's advantages in favor of the Canadian system (see the last column of Parts A and C of Table 6.5).

The same trend can be observed among the American respondents, where the average difference of fourteen percentage points that favored the American health care system before disappears entirely (from 41% to 27% to 35% to 34%; see the last column in Parts B and D of Table 6.5). The advantage of the Canadian system revolves around the question of cost (the gap grows from twenty-six to thirty-five points) and evaluations of the overall performance of the health care system (where it goes from fourteen to twenty-seven points); furthermore, the gap in favor of the US with regard to medication reverses itself in favor of Canada (leading with four points).

The most notable change is in the area of quality of care. The relative advantage of the American health care system, which was distinct when the question was asked from an individual perspective (49% of Americans believed that in this case they would receive the best care in their own country versus 20% who chose Canada), withers away when the question is asked from a collective perspective (35% of Americans surveyed said that Canada would provide the best care for all of their fellow citizens, while 34% said that they would receive better treatment in their own country). These reversals only leave three distinct advantages to the American health care system: quick access to a specialist, quick access to an operating room, and more freedom of choice over one's doctor or hospital.

The data presented in this section allow us to draw a certain number of conclusions about Americans' and Canadians' perceptions of the health care system of their neighboring country. First, Canadians are more willing than Americans to express their opinion about the health care system of their neighboring country. Second, the Canadian health care system is more favorably looked upon by American respondents than the American system is by Canadian respondents. Third, the Canadian health care system largely benefits from a well-known perceived advantage, which is its ability to provide affordable care for everyone. Fourth, the American system does not benefit from a clear single advantage as the Canadian system does. American respondents express different views with regard to the most positive aspect of their health care system, while Canadians largely believe that shorter wait times to see a specialist or have a surgery are the main advantages of the American health care system over their own. Fifth, the question of cost of care (and by extension, of accessibility for all) seems to be a key determinant for respondents in both countries when they are asked to judge health care systems overall. This can explain Canadians' largely negative opinions about the American health care system. This can also explain Americans' generally favorable opinion of the Canadian system. The similar distribution of the variables measuring Americans' impressions of the Canadian health care system and the percentage of them believing that health care costs are more affordable in Canada is remarkable. Close to half of Americans express a favorable opinion about the Canadian health care system (47% positive opinions versus 21% negative opinions and 33% having no opinion; see Table 6.1), which is an amount similar to the percentage of respondents stating that health care costs are more affordable in Canada (49% of respondents versus 23% who believe the opposite and 28% having no opinion; see Table 6.5). Finally, evaluations of a neighboring country's health care system contains a sociotropic dimension that favors the Canadian system, which is largely seen as more equitable, that is, in a better position to ensure quality care for all.

The explanations offered here provide us with some interesting insights that will be examined further with a multivariate model.

CROSS-BORDER PERCEPTIONS: A MULTIVARIATE MODEL

The analyses in this section will revolve around respondents' overall impression of the health care system in the neighboring country as a dependent variable. The explanatory model used will include the five blocks of factors examined in Chapter 5, namely, (1) socioeconomic characteristics, (2) egotropic perceptions, (3) ideological and political preferences, (4) attitudes and opinions about health care systems, (5) sociotropic perceptions (overall judgment of the functioning of the system).

New variables will be added (as a sixth block) to this general model based on the material presented in the previous sections. The first one, called Proplower, is based on the information displayed in Table 6.4. It is coded from a battery of questions asking respondents if the proportion of citizens experiencing specific problems with the health care system (affordability, wait times, etc.) is higher or lower in their own country compared to their neighbor. The two other variables are derived from the information presented in Table 6.5. They are coded from batteries of questions asking respondents which health care system, that of their country or their neighbor, would be the best according to a series of criteria (quality of care, wait times, etc.) for themselves and their family (Bestsystem-IND) or for the population in general (Bestsystem-POP; see the Appendix for more details about the coding of these variables). As in Chapter 5, variables are included in the regression analyses according to the logic of block-recursive estimation. The first model is estimated using only socioeconomic variables, with the other determinants being successively introduced.

A few explanations are in order before examining the determinants of Americans' and Canadians' views about the health care system of their neighboring country. Contrary to the distribution of opinions about one's own health care system, those on the health care system of one's neighboring country are characterized by a high rate of non-response (13% of Canadians surveyed and 33% of Americans surveyed). Given the size of this group, we should first look at the profile of non-respondents before continuing. Regression analyses were carried out by replacing the dependent variable with a dichotomous variable taking the value of 1 in the case of non-response (i.e., "Don't know") and 0 otherwise. All of the independent variables in the model were kept in order to discern the profile of these non-respondents to see if the reluctance to give an opinion on the health care system of a neighboring country was linked to certain political attitudes.

Results of these analyses are presented in Table 6.6. These results are interesting in many ways, and three of them are particularly striking. First, the socioeconomic profile of non-respondents is similar from one country to another and usually corresponds to those who do not express an opinion on political issues (see, notably, Delli Carpini and Keeter 1996; Nadeau, Pétry, and Bélanger 2010). Respondents who are older, less educated, and poorer are less inclined on both sides of the border to express an opinion on the health care system of their neighboring country (women are also less likely to do so in the US). The second interesting result has to do with the large impact of the variable that represents a scale (ProplowerUSA) of questions tapping into the number of Canadian or American citizens worried about certain issues having to do with the health care system (cost, access, wait times, etc.). Results in Table 6.4 have shown that there is a consensus in both countries over the higher number of individuals worried about these questions in the US. Results in Table 6.6 show that those who firmly hold this opinion are also more likely to express an opinion on the overall performance of the health care system of their neighboring country. This result suggests that those who believe that Americans are less worried about their health care system are not as firm in their convictions, since these people largely do not express an opinion on the health care system of their neighboring country.

The last finding that comes out of this analysis of non-respondents has to do with geography and is no less revealing. The rather high rate of non-response in Quebec, where more than 80% of the population is Francophone and may be less exposed to news about the US, is striking. This single variable essentially accounts for the higher level of explained variance in Canada than in the US. To this, the overall higher rate of non-response in the US is added. From this point of view, a model that regroups the data from both countries is particularly interesting. These results first show that the gap between the levels of non-response in both countries is without a doubt statistically significant. The analyses also show that very few variables have a different effect in both countries (very few of the interaction terms included in the model to test this possibility turned out to be

Table 6.6 Determinants of Opinionation in Canada and the US

DV: Opinion	Canada OpinionUSA(CAN)	US OpinionCAN(USA)
AB	1.23*** (0.26)	—
BC	0.87*** (0.24)	—
QC	1.36*** (0.22)	—
Atlantic	0.50 (0.30)	—
Prairies	0.74* (0.31)	—
South	—	–0.03 (0.10)
Male	–0.53*** (0.15)	–0.58*** (0.10)
Age	0.02*** (0.01)	0.01*** (0.00)
Education	–0.16*** (0.05)	–0.14*** (0.04)
Black	—	–0.13 (0.17)
Gvt. emp.	0.26 (0.22)	0.03 (0.22)
Income	–0.09*** (0.03)	–0.04* (0.02)
SatINS	—	0.08 (0.18)
Past2years: egotropic (high)	–0.24 (0.36)	–0.45 (0.28)
Risk scale (high)	–0.57 (0.33)	–0.67*** (0.20)
CANnopid | USAnopid	0.52* (0.20)	0.29* (0.13)
Liberal	–0.04 (0.22)	—
NDP	–0.37 (0.29)	—

(Continued)

Table 6.6 (Continued)

DV: Opinion	Canada OpinionUSA(CAN)	US OpinionCAN(USA)
Bloc	0.25 (0.29)	—
Green	–1.43 (1.37)	—
Democrat	-	0.04 (0.16)
Ideology (right ǀ conservative)	–0.03 (0.42)	0.36 (0.23)
Government role (more)	0.51 (0.30)	0.30 (0.22)
Individualism scale (more)	–0.35 (0.44)	–0.44 (0.28)
Gov. insurance plan	–0.10 (0.08)	–0.08 (0.06)
Universal access	–0.24 (0.29)	0.08 (0.21)
Public system: symbol	–0.11 (0.19)	—
Private system: symbol	—	–0.50*** (0.11)
Health care system: symbol	0.06 (0.17)	–0.09 (0.12)
Past 2 years: sociotropic (high)	0.27 (0.38)	–0.81*** (0.26)
Proplower (USA ǀ CAN)	2.27*** (0.36)	–1.00*** (0.26)
BestsystemIND (USA ǀ CAN)	–0.97* (0.41)	–0.76** (0.29)
BestsystemPOP (USA ǀ CAN)	0.60 (0.40)	–0.30 (0.28)
N	2,414	2,477
Pseudo R^2	0.22	0.13

Notes: Data are weighted. Entries are binary logistic regression coefficients with standard error statistics in parentheses. *$p < 0.05$, **$p < 0.01$, ***$p < 0.001$. Pseudo R^2 are Nagelkerke. For the description of the variables, see the Appendix.

statistically significant). Thus, the conclusion is clear: non-response in the US and Canada with regard to the health care system of the neighboring country arises out of the usual determinants of "opinionation," the particular case of Quebec, and the smaller amount of attention paid to Canadian affairs by Americans.

Another remark is in order before going on to examine the results of the regression analyses and has to do with the previously mentioned inclusion of the three new explanatory factors into the model, namely perceptions on the proportion of citizens worried about health care in the neighboring country and opinions about the system that would be the most advantageous for the respondent and also for all citizens of their country These dimensions are measured with scales constructed from three batteries including six elements in the first set and seven in the other two in order to simplify the analysis and presentation of the results. Before proceeding, it would be helpful to ask if the inclusion of twenty elements corresponding to these three scales would significantly alter the results. Analyses were carried out to determine if this was the case. Two conclusions can be drawn. First, the explanatory performance of the model was affected very little by the inclusion of twenty variables as opposed to the three scales, with the pseudo R^2 values going from 0.298 to 0.302 in the Canadian sample and from 0.106 to 0.114 for the US sample. Secondly, the coefficients for the other variables in the model remained practically the same from one operationalization to another. Thirdly, given the strong correlations between some of these variables, about a quarter of them (eleven out of forty) remained statistically significant once they were included into the analysis. Among them, the nature of the variables exercising the most impact is revealing. The influential variables are those that have to do with the number of citizens worried about the cost of health care and the system that would best "guarantee" affordable health care for everyone (i.e., "comprehensive, guaranteed and affordable insurance plan covering their health care needs"). These results confirm the importance of cost and coverage in the evaluation of health care systems and strongly suggest that the introduction of the three scales into the model will reflect this importance.

Results of the regression analyses are presented in Tables 6.7 and 6.8. The overall performance of the model differs from country to country, relatively weak in Canada (pseudo R^2 of 0.24) and much better in the US (pseudo R^2 of 0.57). How can we explain this? There can be two main reasons. The first concerns the distribution of the dependent variable, which is much more asymmetrical in Canada. The second, which we will explore in greater detail, has to do with the structure of US public opinion on questions of health care.

The first observation about Americans' and Canadians' viewpoints has to do with different cleavages conditioning opinions regarding the health care system of their neighboring country. Canadians who have a more favorable view of the American system are Quebecers, men, and those with a high income (surprisingly, Albertans seem to have a more negative opinion of the American system). The picture is different in the US, where opinions about the Canadian health care system are more negative among those living in the South, older respondents, and respondents with a higher income (see column 1 of Tables 6.7 and 6.8). Thus, income plays a different role depending on the country. Wealthier Canadians have a more favorable opinion of the American system while wealthier Americans have a more negative opinion of the Canadian system. Another significant result is the very favorable opinion of African Americans toward the Canadian system. Finally, while education does not have an effect on Canadians' opinions, it is associated with more favorable opinions among Americans toward the Canadian system.

Overall, the explanatory power of socioeconomic variables remains weak. What about the variables that reflect respondents' direct experiences with the health care system? Our expectation was that the impact of these considerations will be smaller on respondents' cross-border perceptions than on their opinion about their own health care system. The results confirm this hypothesis (see column 2 in Tables 6.7 and 6.8). The effect of retrospective egotropic perceptions on cross-border perceptions is significant for Canadians only: a positive judgment about the medical care received in the past is negatively related with opinions about the health care system of the US (–0.66). But this association is much weaker than for respondents' satisfaction with the Canadian health care system (the value for the coefficient is 3.93; see Table 5.2, column 2). The results are somewhat different concerning the risk scale. Being worried about getting quality health care in the future has no impact on Canadians' opinion about the US health care system but is strongly linked to Americans' views about the Canadian system (coefficients of –0.06, not significant, and 0.75, significant, for Canada and the US, respectively). This finding reinforces the notion that positive views about the Canadian health care system in the US are linked to the perception that this system, thanks to its universal character, offers individuals more security and predictability concerning the quality of the care that will be received in the future. It is interesting to note in this perspective that those who do not experience this problem of accessibility in an acute fashion—for example, those who are more satisfied with their health insurance plan—tend to view the Canadian system in a more negative light (the coefficient for this variable is negative at –0.53 and statistically significant; see Table 6.8, column 2). That being said, the main conclusion remains. The overall contribution of personal experiences with the health care system is relatively limited as testified by the small shift in the pseudo R^2 in both countries when this block of variables is introduced as compared to what was observed in our previous chapter with perceptions about the national health care system.

What about the variables that reflect respondents' partisan and ideological preferences? The results are presented in columns 3 and 4 of Tables 6.7 and 6.8. Those that deal with more general preferences (column 3) are

Table 6.7 Opinion about the American Health Care System (Evaluation: Neighbor)

DV: OpinionUSA(CAN)	Model 1	Model 2	Model 3	Model 4	Model 5	Model 6
AB	–0.32* (0.14)	–0.35* (0.14)	–0.47*** (0.15)	–0.47** (0.15)	–0.47** (0.15)	–0.41** (0.15)
BC	–0.21 (0.12)	–0.21 (0.13)	–0.23 (0.13)	–0.24 (0.13)	–0.27* (0.14)	–0.21 (0.14)
QC	0.38*** (0.10)	0.35** (0.11)	0.42*** (0.13)	0.22 (0.13)	0.22 (0.13)	0.03 (0.14)
Atlantic	0.24 (0.15)	0.32* (0.16)	0.47** (0.17)	0.54*** (0.17)	0.53** (0.17)	0.54** (0.17)
Prairies	–0.02 (0.16)	0.08 (0.18)	0.08 (0.18)	0.02 (0.18)	0.02 (0.18)	–0.01 (0.19)
Male	0.24** (0.08)	0.23** (0.08)	0.06 (0.09)	0.09 (0.09)	0.10 (0.09)	0.07 (0.09)
Age	–0.00 (0.00)	0.00 (0.00)	–0.00 (0.00)	0.00 (0.00)	0.00 (0.00)	0.00 (0.00)
Education	–0.03 (0.02)	–0.01 (0.03)	0.04 (0.03)	0.04 (0.03)	0.05 (0.03)	0.05 (0.03)
Gvt. emp.	–0.08 (0.12)	–0.08 (0.13)	–0.11 (0.13)	–0.11 (0.13)	–0.13 (0.13)	–0.15 (0.13)
Income	0.04*** (0.01)	0.05*** (0.01)	0.02 (0.01)	0.03 (0.01)	0.02 (0.01)	0.02 (0.01)
Past2years: egotropic (high)		–0.66*** (0.20)	–0.62** (0.21)	–0.25 (0.21)	–0.37 (0.22)	–0.08 (0.22)
Risk scale (high)		–0.06 (0.18)	–0.07 (0.18)	–0.04 (0.18)	0.03 (0.19)	–0.64** (0.20)
CANnopid			–0.26* (0.13)	–0.28* (0.13)	–0.28* (0.13)	–0.23 (0.13)
Liberal			–0.21 (0.12)	–0.08 (0.12)	–0.08 (0.12)	–0.07 (0.12)
NDP			–0.23 (0.15)	–0.20 (0.15)	–0.20 (0.15)	–0.16 (0.16)
Bloc			0.01 (0.20)	–0.06 (0.21)	–0.04 (0.21)	0.03 (0.21)
Green			–0.44 (0.41)	–0.31 (0.42)	–0.27 (0.43)	–0.28 (0.43)

DV: OpinionUSA(CAN)	Model 1	Model 2	Model 3	Model 4	Model 5	Model 6
Ideology (right)			1.41*** (0.22)	1.05*** (0.23)	0.99*** (0.23)	0.78*** (0.24)
Government role (more)			–0.26 (0.18)	0.08 (0.18)	0.06 (0.18)	0.12 (0.19)
Individualism scale (more)			1.42*** (0.25)	0.73** (0.25)	0.76** (0.26)	0.66** (0.26)
Gov. insurance plan				–0.13* (0.05)	–0.14* (0.05)	–0.12* (0.06)
Universal access				–1.16*** (0.19)	–1.20*** (0.19)	–1.12*** (0.20)
Public system: symbol				–0.24 (0.13)	–0.23 (0.13)	–0.04 (0.13)
Health care system: symbol				–0.53*** (0.11)	–0.51*** (0.11)	–0.43*** (0.11)
Past2years: sociotropic (high)					0.30 (0.24)	0.60* (0.24)
Proplower (USA)						1.88*** (0.25)
BestsystemIND (USA)						0.58* (0.23)
BestsystemPOP (USA)						0.87*** (0.23)
Cut 1 (constant)	–0.34 (0.19)	–0.61 (0.27)	0.27 (0.36)	–1.34*** (0.39)	–1.31*** (0.41)	–0.11 (0.43)
Cut 2 (constant)	1.85*** (0.20)	1.59*** (0.27)	2.61*** (0.36)	1.13** (0.39)	1.18** (0.41)	2.48*** (0.43)
Cut 3 (constant)	3.70*** (0.22)	3.41*** (0.29)	4.49*** (0.38)	3.01*** (0.40)	3.17*** (0.42)	4.56*** (0.45)
N	2,480	2,167	2,167	2,167	2,133	2,133
Pseudo R^2	0.03	0.03	0.11	0.18	0.19	0.24

Notes: Data are weighted. Entries are ordered logistic regression coefficients with standard errors in parentheses. Pseudo R^2 are Nagelkerke. $^{*}p < 0.05$, $^{**}p < 0.01$, $^{***}p < 0.001$. For the description of the variables, see the Appendix.

Table 6.8 Opinion about the Canadian Health Care System (Evaluation: Neighbor)

DV: OpinionCAN(USA)	Model 1	Model 2	Model 3	Model 4	Model 5	Model 6
South	–0.20*	–0.23*	–0.11	–0.16	–0.18	–0.15
	(0.08)	(0.09)	(0.10)	(0.10)	(0.10)	(0.10)
Male	–0.04	–0.02	0.07	0.09	0.10	0.10
	(0.08)	(0.09)	(0.09)	(0.10)	(0.10)	(0.10)
Age	–0.02***	–0.02***	–0.01***	–0.02***	–0.02***	–0.01***
	(0.00)	(0.00)	(0.00)	(0.00)	(0.00)	(0.00)
Education	0.06*	0.05	–0.00	0.00	0.01	–0.01
	(0.03)	(0.03)	(0.03)	(0.04)	(0.04)	(0.04)
Black	0.86***	0.79***	0.27	0.33*	0.36*	0.49**
	(0.12)	(0.14)	(0.15)	(0.15)	(0.16)	(0.16)
Gvt. emp.	–0.02	–0.05	–0.02	–0.07	–0.07	–0.01
	(0.18)	(0.19)	(0.20)	(0.20)	(0.20)	(0.21)
Income	–0.04***	–0.02	0.01	0.02	0.02	0.01
	(0.01)	(0.01)	(0.02)	(0.02)	(0.02)	(0.02)
SatINS		–0.53***	–0.24	0.01	0.00	0.24
		(0.15)	(0.16)	(0.17)	(0.17)	(0.18)
Past2years: egotropic (high)		–0.18	0.35	0.40	0.39	0.78**
		(0.25)	(0.26)	(0.27)	(0.28)	(0.29)
Risk scale (high)		0.75***	0.48**	0.14	0.15	–0.22
		(0.17)	(0.18)	(0.18)	(0.19)	(0.20)
USAnopid			0.23	0.16	0.14	0.04
			(0.13)	(0.13)	(0.13)	(0.13)
Democrat			0.42**	0.34*	0.31*	0.14
			(0.14)	(0.15)	(0.15)	(0.15)
Ideology (conservative)			–1.71***	–1.12***	–1.10***	–0.88***
			(0.21)	(0.22)	(0.22)	(0.23)
Government role (more)			1.57***	0.59**	0.59**	0.54**
			(0.19)	(0.20)	(0.20)	(0.21)
Individualism scale (more)			–2.00***	–0.75**	–0.77**	–0.28
			(0.25)	(0.26)	(0.26)	(0.28)
Gov. insurance plan				0.56***	0.55***	0.45***
				(0.06)	(0.06)	(0.06)
Universal access				1.25***	1.25***	0.92***
				(0.20)	(0.20)	(0.21)

DV: OpinionCAN(USA)	Model 1	Model 2	Model 3	Model 4	Model 5	Model 6
Private system: symbol				–0.11 (0.11)	–0.10 (0.11)	0.12 (0.11)
Health care system: symbol				0.25* (0.11)	0.26* (0.11)	0.49*** (0.11)
Past2years: sociotropic (high)					0.02 (0.24)	0.54* (0.25)
Proplower (CAN)						2.00*** (0.26)
BestsystemIND (CAN)						2.05*** (0.28)
BestsystemPOP (CAN)						0.76** (0.27)
Cut 1 (constant)	–2.97*** (0.22)	–2.90*** (0.31)	–3.91*** (0.41)	–2.16*** (0.43)	–2.12*** (0.44)	0.67 (0.49)
Cut 2 (constant)	–1.66*** (0.21)	–1.51*** (0.30)	–2.15*** (0.40)	–0.24 (0.43)	–0.19 (0.43)	2.90*** (0.49)
Cut 3 (constant)	0.49* (0.21)	0.79* (0.30)	0.65 (0.40)	2.92*** (0.43)	2.96*** (0.44)	6.54*** (0.51)
N	2,258	1,860	1,860	1,860	1,834	1,834
Pseudo R^2	0.06	0.09	0.37	0.46	0.46	0.57

Notes: Data are weighted. Entries are ordered logistic regression coefficients with standard errors in parentheses. Pseudo R^2 are Nagelkerke. $*p < 0.05$, $**p < 0.01$, $***p < 0.001$. For the description of the variables, see the Appendix.

both interesting and revealing. Variables measuring general preferences have much more of an impact in the US than in Canada: adding them to the model's estimation increases the pseudo R^2 from 0.09 to 0.37 in the first case and from 0.03 to 0.11 in the second. These figures show that Americans are much more divided, and along much more clear ideological lines, than Canadians are regarding the presumed pluses and minuses of the health care system of their neighboring country.

The overall consistency of the results is also striking. In Canada, the least favorable opinions toward the American health care system are seen among ideological groups (more left-wing, interventionists, less individualistic) and partisans (Liberals, New Democrats) that support a larger role for the public sector, while the opposite is true in the US, where Democrats, liberals, those who favor a larger role for the state, and those scoring low on individualism express the most favorable opinions toward the Canadian health care system.

What about the effect of preferences more directly related to the issue of health care, which constitute our fourth block of explanatory variables? The results are also very clear in this case; their explanatory power is larger in the American case (raising the pseudo R^2 from 0.37 to 0.46) than in Canada (increase from 0.11 to 0.18), which is in line with aforementioned expectations regarding more pronounced cueing and priming effects in the US. The consistency of the results is also obvious. Canadians favoring strong public intervention in health care have a very negative opinion of the American system, while on the contrary the same people in the US have a very positive opinion of the Canadian system (for example, note the opposite signs for the statistically significant variables "government insurance plan" and "universal access" in column 4).

An important question for understanding the formation of opinion toward health care is establishing whether or not respondents are using global evaluations of their own health care system to form their opinion about the health care system in the neighboring country. In other words, does Canadians' assessment about the recent performance of their own health care system make them more likely to have a favorable opinion toward the American system and vice versa? The answer to this question is provided by the results in column 5. The results are clear. Americans' and Canadians' overall assessments about the evolution of the quality of health care in their country only very marginally influences their opinion of the system in the neighboring country. The change in the pseudo R^2 in both countries is negligible and the variables measuring these sociotropic perceptions are not significant in both cases. This finding is in line with our previous result showing that direct experience (i.e., egotropic perceptions) are weakly linked to cross-border perceptions. Overall, these results reinforce the idea that cross-border perceptions result from a mix of information and predispositions.

Finally, what about respondents' direct comparisons between the American and Canadian systems? As previously mentioned, three scales were constructed to answer this question (see the Appendix for a detailed description). The first asked respondents whether the proportion of the population who have difficulty getting access to health care (because of cost, wait times, inability to receive proper medication, etc.) is higher in Canada or in the US for the Canadian respondents and vice versa in the US. A high score on this scale should therefore be associated with a negative evaluation of the national health care system and a positive assessment of the neighboring country's system. The second scale asked respondents in which country (his own or that of the neighboring country) they would be in the best position to receive the best care if they became ill. The scale was coded so the sign attached to it should again be negative for respondents' own health care system and positive for that of the neighboring country. The question that asked in which country the entire population (and not the respondent in particular) would be more likely to obtain the best care in case of illness is coded in the same fashion.

The results obtained when adding these variables as a sixth and last block are presented in column 6. In examining the tables, three things stand out. Once again, the overall performance of this group of variables is more striking in the US than in Canada (increases in the pseudo R^2 of 0.11 and 0.05 for the US and Canada, respectively). The consistency of the results is impressive: the three variables corresponding to this block of variables are all of the expected sign (positive for both countries) and statistically significant. The fact that both egotropic comparisons, which lead the individual to choose the health care system that would be the most beneficial to them, and sociotropic comparisons, which press the respondent to choose the system that would be best for the entire population, are significant constitutes an undeniably interesting theoretical finding because it shows that individuals take into account these two dimensions when evaluating a health care system. That said, the fact that the impact of the egotropic dimension is roughly three times as important in the US (coefficient of 2.05) as in Canada (0.58) neatly confirms that individualistic values in the US (McClosky and Zaller 1984; Zaller and Feldman 1992) not only color perceptions about the US health care system but assessments about the Canadian system as well.

To round up the presentation, we now turn our attention to the changes in probabilities displayed in Tables 6.9 and 6.10. Given the small proportion of Canadians with positive views about the American health care system, the changes computed represent the probability of expressing a very positive opinion of the Canadian system (very positive) and a positive opinion of the American system (positive or very positive). A look at the results confirms that all the substantive findings discussed in this chapter are confirmed. The larger impact of partisan and ideological preferences in the US, either general or issue-specific, is particularly striking. The modest contribution of respondents' assessments of the performance of their own health care system on their cross-border perceptions also stands out. Finally, the contrast between the profiles of those holding positive views of the neighboring health care system is remarkable. One of the most telling results in this regard is the opposite impact of individualism in both samples. Americans with individualistic views strongly dislike the Canadian health care system whereas Canadians sharing the same anti-collectivist attitudes tend, to the contrary, to strongly like the American health care system.

Table 6.9 Change in Probabilities Related to the Opinion about the American Health Care System (Evaluation: Neighbor)

DV: OpinionUSA(CAN)	Model 1	Model 2	Model 3	Model 4	Model 5	Model 6
AB	–0.03	–0.04	–0.05	–0.04	–0.04	–0.04
BC	–0.02	–0.02	–0.02	–0.02	–0.03	–0.02
QC	0.04	0.04	0.04	0.02	0.02	0.00
Atlantic	0.03	0.03	0.04	0.05	0.05	0.05
Prairies	–0.00	0.00	0.01	0.00	0.00	–0.00
Male	0.02	0.02	0.01	0.01	0.01	0.01
Age	–0.000	0.000	–0.000	0.000	0.000	0.000
Education	–0.00	–0.00	0.00	0.00	0.00	0.01
Gvt. emp.	–0.00	–0.01	–0.01	–0.01	–0.01	–0.01
Income	0.004	0.005	0.002	0.002	0.002	0.002
Past2years: egotropic (high)		–0.07	–0.06	–0.02	–0.03	–0.01
Risk scale (high)		–0.01	–0.01	–0.00	0.00	0.06
CANnopid			–0.03	–0.03	–0.03	–0.02
Liberal			–0.02	–0.01	–0.01	–0.01
NDP			–0.02	–0.02	–0.02	–0.01
Bloc			0.00	–0.01	–0.00	0.00
Green			–0.04	–0.03	–0.03	–0.03
Ideology (right)			0.14	0.10	0.09	0.07
Government role (more)			–0.03	0.01	0.01	0.01
Individualism scale (more)			0.14	0.07	0.07	0.06
Gov. insurance plan				–0.01	–0.01	–0.01
Universal access				–0.11	–0.11	–0.10
Public system: symbol				–0.02	–0.02	–0.00
Health care system: symbol				–0.05	–0.05	–0.04
Past2years: sociotropic (high)					0.03	0.05
Proplower (USA)						0.17
BestsystemIND (USA)						0.05
BestsystemPOP (USA)						0.08

Notes: Entries in the table are the changes in probability that the dependent variable takes its highest value (very positive or moderately positive) when an explanatory variable varies from its minimum to its maximum value. All calculations were performed with Stata 11.0.

Table 6.10 Change in Probabilities Related to the Opinion about the Canadian Health Care System (Evaluation: Neighbor)

DV: OpinionCAN(USA)	Model 1	Model 2	Model 3	Model 4	Model 5	Model 6
South	−0.03	−0.04	−0.02	−0.02	−0.02	−0.02
Male	−0.01	−0.00	0.01	0.01	0.01	0.01
Age	−0.003	−0.003	−0.002	−0.002	−0.002	−0.001
Education	0.01	0.01	−0.00	0.00	0.00	−0.00
Black	0.15	0.14	0.04	0.05	0.05	0.06
Gvt. emp.	−0.00	−0.01	−0.00	−0.01	−0.01	−0.00
Income	−0.007	−0.003	0.002	0.003	0.003	0.002
SatINS		−0.09	−0.04	0.00	0.00	0.03
Past2years: egotropic (high)		−0.03	0.05	0.05	0.05	0.10
Risk scale (high)		0.13	0.07	0.02	0.02	−0.03
USAnopid			0.03	0.02	0.02	0.00
Democrat			0.06	0.05	0.04	0.02
Ideology (conservative)			−0.25	−0.15	−0.15	−0.11
Government role (more)			0.23	0.08	0.08	0.07
Individualism scale (more)			−0.29	−0.10	−0.10	−0.03
Gov. insurance plan				0.08	0.08	0.05
Universal access				0.17	0.17	0.11
Private system: symbol				−0.01	−0.01	0.01
Health care system: symbol				0.03	0.03	0.06
Past2years: sociotropic (high)					−0.00	0.07
Proplower (CAN)						0.24
BestsystemIND (CAN)						0.25
BestsystemPOP (CAN)						0.09

Notes: Entries in the table are the changes in probability that the dependent variable takes its highest value (very positive) when an explanatory variable varies from its minimum to its maximum value. All calculations were performed with Stata 11.0.

CONCLUSION

Many interesting conclusions can be drawn from the examination of Americans' and Canadians' cross-border perceptions of the health care system of their neighboring country. First, these results suggest that cross-border perceptions of health care systems can be explained by the circulation of factual information about the topic in question. The average profile of survey respondents who did not express an opinion on this public policy is the same as those who did not express an opinion on the health care system of the neighboring country. In addition to these standard characteristics (e.g., lower education and lower income), two factors more specific to our study can be added to our research question. The higher rate of nonresponse among Francophone Quebecers and Americans in general could be explained by linguistic reasons in the first case and less visibility of Canadian health issues in the US in the second case. These results suggest that Canadians' opinions about the American health care system (as well as Americans' opinions about the Canadian health care system) are not entirely artificial and at least rest in part on factual knowledge.

The portrait of cross-border perceptions that emerges from this analysis is clear: Canadians largely have a negative opinion of the American health care system while Americans have a more positive view of the Canadian system. These overall impressions rest on well-entrenched perceptions about both systems. In the eyes of survey respondents from both countries, the main advantage of the Canadian health care system is its affordable care and universal coverage. Opinions on the strengths of the American health care system are less consensual. The possibility of quicker access to care and greater freedom of choice over one's doctor or hospital tend to be seen as distinctive advantages of the American system.

This configuration of opinions on specific aspects of health care systems and overall impressions on how well they function tends to show that respondents privilege concerns of cost and access to care in their evaluations of health care systems. It also shows that respondents base their judgments of the performance of health care systems on both egotropic and sociotropic considerations. Of note, the advantage of the Canadian system seems to become more pronounced when placed in a collective frame—that is, when respondents are asked to evaluate the advantages for all their country's citizens and not just for themselves individually.

These cross-border opinions also seem to be explained by the place that American and Canadian systems have in the debates over health care reform on both sides of the border. Debates over the merits and drawbacks of both countries' health care systems have crystallized around two distinct images that have become decisional shortcuts that citizens in both countries have used to form an opinion of their neighboring country's health care system: that of "socialized medicine" in Canada and of a "two-tier" system in the US (Marmor 1993; Nadeau et al. 2010). Notice that the frame used in the

US is more *partisan oriented,* whereas the frame used in the Canadian debate instead refers to notions of *equality.*

These images have been perpetuated by camps in both countries either favoring change or advocating the status quo. Moreover, these camps belong to different ideological families, depending on the country. While more leftist political forces want to preserve the integrity of the Canadian health care system, the same forces are trying to change their system south of the border. At the heart of these debates lies the issue of the place of the private and public sectors in health care provision. "Conservatives" on both sides advocate a larger role for the private sector in health care delivery in order for it to grow in Canada and be maintained in the US. On the other hand, "liberals" in the US and Canada want the public sector to be a key actor in the health care system and therefore prefer that its role be maintained in Canada and increased in the US.

Partisans of reform in the US emphasize the equitable nature of the Canadian system while their opponents underscore the long wait times and less freedom of choice that also characterizes it. Proponents of change in Canada often invoke the efficiency and greater flexibility of the American health care system brought about by the larger presence of the private sector in the delivery of health care in the US. Defenders of the public system in Canada focus on showing that an American-style system would create two categories of citizens: richer citizens who would have adequate coverage and the less fortunate citizens who would not have access to high-quality care.

All of these findings help us understand the nature and impact of survey respondents' socioeconomic profiles and personal experience, as well as partisan and ideological preferences, on opinions of their neighboring country's health care system. While less wealthy and leftist respondents in Canada have a negative opinion of the American health care system, people having the same profile have a favorable opinion of the Canadian health care system. What is even more important is perhaps the fact that Americans' partisan preferences influence their opinions on the Canadian health care system more so than the opposite. This finding shows a greater amount of polarization in the US than in Canada over the issue of health care. Without a doubt, this phenomenon can be explained by a "priming effect" due to the fact that the US just had a fierce debate over health care reform. In the eyes of some, the debate still is not over in the US. However, our results show that health care is a valence issue in Canada and a positional issue in the US.

In his recent work, Larry Bartels (2008) claimed that Americans' ideological predispositions weighed heavily on their opinions on public policy, even if it was against their own interests. The findings of this chapter clearly illustrate this dynamic. The formula "politics is in the way" seems to apply more to Americans' opinions on the Canadian health care system than the opposite. We now turn in Chapter 7 to whether these cross-border perceptions have an influence on Americans' and Canadians' inclinations to support changes to their own health care system.

7 An Explanatory Model of Opinion toward Health Care Reform

The natural starting point for a study of citizens' perceptions and opinions of their own health system is to explore whether these attitudes are related to (accurate) views of the way the system works. The logical ending point is to examine whether these attitudes translate into policy outcomes—whether they point toward, and inform, changes in health care policy. One aim of this penultimate chapter is to understand the factors that motivate Americans and Canadians to support the idea of reforming their health care system in meaningful ways.

There are good reasons to believe that public opinion will structure policy change. The very importance of health care as an issue suggests that citizens will be attentive to the debate on health care reform. The importance of this same issue for governments and society in general also suggests that discussions of possible reforms will generate media interest, with political parties and numerous advocacy groups becoming interested as well (Jacobs and Shapiro 2000; Soroka, Maioni, and Martin 2013). The intensity of the debate over health care and voter interest in this issue suggest that citizens' views on health care reform will be firmer and more consistent than those on matters of lesser importance; and that governments have an unusually strong incentive to pay attention to public preferences on this issue.

Previous chapters have looked at attitudes toward existing health care systems. This chapter focuses on attitudes about reform. It is divided into four parts. We will first briefly discuss the factors that may be influential in driving someone to support or reject health care reforms. We will examine the impact of some of these determinants in a descriptive fashion. A multivariate model will then be used to assess the impact of these various factors, all things being equal. A brief conclusion will follow.

THE DETERMINANTS OF DEMAND FOR HEALTH CARE REFORM IN THE US AND CANADA

Results from previous chapters suggest several factors that might lead a citizen to demand health care reforms. One hypothesis states that one's own direct experience with the health care system will affect their evaluation of it and consequently affect one's propensity to demand change. An individual's demographic profile can be seen as indicative of one's relationship to the health system and could be linked to their opinion on changing it. Work in both Canada and the United States (Soroka et al. 2013; Gelman, Lee, and Ghitza 2010) has shown that older people, who are more dependent on the health system, are also the most likely to want reform. Access to health care is also linked to a person's socioeconomic status. It is therefore possible to argue that poorer people are more likely to support reforms that would extend health care coverage to the greatest number of people. Finally, performance of one's own health system may vary from one region to another; therefore, we might be able to observe regional variation in the appetite for reform.

What this suggests is that an individual's profile provides us with a set of indicators about their experience with the health care system, and that these same indicators can be connected to how much they support health care reform. That said, first-hand experience with and perceptions of the health care system are more direct and meaningful indicators. These perceptions, of an egotropic nature, can be either retrospective or prospective, as we have seen in previous chapters. The egotropic and retrospective variable used in this book measures an individual's perception about the quality of care received in the past two years. The theoretical expectation in this case is clear: a significant negative relationship should be seen between the quality of care received in the past and support for a reform of the health system. In the same fashion, a person satisfied with his or her health insurance plan in the US should be less inclined to support reform of the health care system.

A person's past experiences, their present situation (e.g., socioeconomic status), and the current debate over the health care system ought to influence their expectations about the system's future performance. These expectations measure the probability that an individual will receive the same quality of health care in the future, or in other words, the amount of risk that they might not be provided with the same quality of care in the future. Three theoretical expectations can be drawn from this statement. First, a positive and significant link should exist between the level of anticipated risk and willingness to reform the system. Such perceptions, both egotropic and prospective, should exert a greater impact on a person's support for reform than their past experience does. Additionally, reforms focus on the future performance of a health care system. Quality of care received in the past is an indicator, but does not necessarily provide a guarantee about what the quality and accessibility of health care will be like in the future. It is possible that good health care system performance in the past may be impaired by reforms. This is why prospective assessments should play a larger role than retrospective perceptions in determining support for reform.

The third and final expectation follows from the first two: an analysis of the debates over health care shows that discussions in Canada focused significantly more on a frame that gave a greater weight to prospective assessments than debates in the US did. This framing suggests that an aging population and lack of resources will not allow for the same quality of care that Canadians have received in the past. In other words, the ideals of universality and broad coverage needs will come under severe strain in the future. This interpretation is consistent with the idea that Canadians can be simultaneously satisfied with the level of care they receive at the moment and concerned about the care that they may receive in the future. This way of characterizing the debate over health care reform is less present in the US; therefore it is reasonable to believe that concerns about the sustainability of one's health system in the long term, particularly with respect to its ability to provide wide-ranging and high-quality health services, will be more pronounced in Canada than in its neighboring country.

Other factors that might affect support for health care reform are threefold. We can expect that perceptions about recent developments in the quality of health care in general (and not specifically about that received by individuals) are strongly and negatively related to demand for reform. A person who believes that health care has generally improved in recent years will be much less inclined to believe that reform is needed.

Political attitudes in general and opinions on the optimal functioning of the health care system are also likely to play a role in a person's demand for health care reform. However, their impact is likely to be different in the US and Canada. First, this difference should be seen in the direction of the effects. While health care system reform in Canada is widely seen as meaning a bigger role for the private sector, it means the opposite in the US. Thus, in the Canadian case, the word "reform" is associated with privatization, while in the US it is associated with state intervention. Given this context, it is expected that conservative attitudes, generally less favorable to the state, will be positively related to support for health care reform in Canada and negatively related to reform in the US.

Attitudes and perceptions of the demand for reforms should vary in intensity between the two countries. In Canada, the debate over health care reform peaked in the early 2000s and has since resurfaced sporadically, without reaching the intensity that characterized the debate some ten years ago. This has helped depolarize the debate and accentuate the "valence" nature of this issue in Canada. Obviously, the situation is radically different in the US, where health care reform has sparked intense and polarized debate largely centered on partisan and ideological lines. Therefore, we can expect that general political attitudes and opinions more specific to the functioning of the health system are more directly related to the demand for reform in the US than in Canada. However, we also expect one exception to appear with regard to the symbolic value of the health care system in both countries: strong in Canada and much less intense in the US. This would suggest that the link between perceptions about the system and support for reforms will be stronger in Canada than in the US.

THE DEMAND FOR REFORMS: A FIRST LOOK

We will now examine the determinants of support for health care system reform in the US and Canada. Our analysis will first be descriptive before moving on to a discussion of our multivariate models. The question used to measure the willingness of respondents to seek changes to their health care system is the same used for the Commonwealth Fund International Health Policy Survey and reads as follows: "What approach would you say that this country's health system requires at present: a full rebuilding from the ground up, some fairly major repairs, some minor tuning up, or everything is fine the way it is?"

The answers to this question for the US and Canada have already been presented in Chapter 1. The results are very similar to those obtained in recent versions of the Commonwealth Policy Survey: the number of respondents refusing to give an answer is very low and the appetite for reform is greater in the US than in Canada. In fact, while one in five Americans wants a complete transformation of the health system, this proportion is only 8% in Canada. Similarly, while nearly two in five Canadians want only minor changes to their health care system (39%), this percentage is only 26% in the US. This result is not surprising. Data from the previous chapters have shown that Americans are less satisfied with their health system than Canadians are. Therefore, it is consistent that they are more likely to seek (or support) reform.

Actually, the differences observed between the US and Canada were more pronounced in the past. A brief look at the evolution of public opinion in both countries reveals partial convergence over time. For example, in 1988, 56% of Canadians wanted only minor changes to their health care system, with 38% opting for major changes and only 5% for a complete transformation. However, this high level of satisfaction would not continue for very long. Ten years later, Canadians' pessimism about their health system peaked. Only 20% wanted just minor changes, whereas 56% supported radical changes and 23% advocated a top-to-bottom overhaul of the system. Canadian public opinion has varied considerably over the past quarter century with regard to health care system reform. Optimistic and satisfied at the end of the 1980s, Canadians had become pessimistic and unhappy during the 1990s, but a certain optimism can be seen again in recent years (see Mendelsohn 2002; Soroka et al. 2013).

The situation has developed differently in the US. In 1988, barely 10% of Americans wanted minor changes to their health care system, 60% favored major changes, and 29% demanded a complete transformation. Nearly twenty years later, in 2007, the figures had changed little. There were now 16% who wanted only minor changes, 48% who opted for radical change, and 34% who claimed to want a major revamping of the health system. The figures for the 2010 Commonwealth Survey (29%, 41%, and 27%) and those of our own study (20%, 49%, and 26%) continue to highlight Americans' stronger desire for change when compared to Canadians. However, we can no longer speak of a massive difference between citizens of both countries on this question. Americans and Canadians seemed to live in parallel universes in the late 1980s, with the former requesting altogether cosmetic changes to their health system and the latter instead wanting a radical transformation. This discrepancy was considerably reduced in the 1990s, and the rift in public opinion between both countries has not reappeared since (although a gap still exists). It is against this backdrop that we will now examine the factors related to the demand for reform in the two countries.

The list of factors that will be examined overlap with the determinants of satisfaction with the performance of the health system discussed previously. For example, willingness to demand reform may depend on the performance of the health care system in a given area. One of the most marked divisions in this regard is that between Quebec residents relative to other Canadians, no less than 81% of the Quebec residents surveyed demanded profound changes in the health system, a proportion almost thirty percentage points higher than anywhere else in the country. This perception about the particular challenges of the Quebec health system seems to be shared by health professionals in the province. A Commonwealth Fund survey conducted in 2012 and published in 2013 shows that the percentage of Quebec physicians who felt that the health care system in their province was working properly is not only the lowest in Canada, but also the lowest when compared to ten industrialized countries (Commonwealth Fund 2013).

The appetite for reform is not only related to the quality of care received by individuals in the past but also their degree of confidence in the quality of care they will receive in the future. Table 7.1 illustrates these relationships. In both the US and Canada, those who are the most satisfied with the quality of care (Panel A of the table) and more optimistic about maintaining said quality in the future (Panel B of the table) are also those who are less likely to demand health reform. The most interesting piece of data from this table comes from the influence of prospective and retrospective assessments. In

Table 7.1 Perceptions of Health Care Received and to Be Received and Support for Health Care Reforms in Canada and the US

Panel A. Evaluation of the Medical Care Received in the Past Two Years

	Canada			
Health Care Received	***Minor Changes***	***Major Changes***	***Completely Rebuilt***	**%**
Very poor	10	65	25	2
Poor	21	61	19	4
Fair	32	58	9	28
Very good	44	50	6	47
Excellent	54	39	8	19

US				
Health Care Received	*Minor Changes*	*Major Changes*	*Completely Rebuilt*	%
Very poor	9	28	63	1
Poor	18	46	37	3
Fair	19	55	27	30
Very good	31	52	16	49
Excellent	41	42	17	17

Panel B. Expectations About Risk of Not Getting High-Quality Medical Care in the Future

Canada				
Risk Level	*Minor Changes*	*Major hanges*	*Completely Rebuilt*	%
Very high	17	63	20	16
High	29	61	10	31
Low	48	48	4	38
Very low	70	25	5	15

US				
Risk Level	*Minor Changes*	*Major Changes*	*Completely Rebuilt*	%
Very high	15	45	40	23
High	23	57	19	32
Low	33	53	13	28
Very low	47	43	10	16

Notes: Sample sizes are 3,522 and 3,542 for Canada and the US, respectively (DKs are excluded). Data are weighted.
Panel A: CANADA: $\chi 2 = 173.65$, $p < 0.000$ with 8 df; Cramer's V = 0.16; Kendall's Tau-B = –0.18, $p < 0.000$.
Panel A: USA: $\chi 2 = 182.22$, $p < 0.000$ with 8 df; Cramer's V = 0.16; Kendall's Tau-B = –0.18, $p < 0.000$.
Panel B: CANADA: $\chi 2 = 398.03$, $p < 0.000$ with 6 df; Cramer's V = 0.26; Kendall's Tau-B = –0.32, $p < 0.000$.
Panel B: USA: $\chi 2 = 301.94$, $p < 0.000$ with 6 df; Cramer's V = 0.23; Kendall's Tau-B = –0.26, $p < 0.000$.
Question Wording: *"Health Care Received" Variable:* Overall, how do you rate the quality of medical care that you and your family have received in the past 2 years? *"Risk" Variable:* The "risk" variable comprised a series of variables asking about the risks that in the coming years a respondent or his/her family will be unable to afford needed health care, get the most effective drugs, received high-quality health care, or wait longer than reasonable to get health care services (scale recoded from very high to very low risk; categories correspond to following values: very high, 0–0.25; high, 0.33–0.50; low, 0.58–0.75; very low, 0.83–1.0; tau-c is calculated from the original scale). Percentages under the column % represent the proportion of the sample in each category for the "quality" and "risk" variable. Other entries represent the percentages of respondents supporting health care reform for each level of satisfaction with health care received in the past or risk level about not high-quality health care in the future.

both countries, expectations about the future quality of health care (tau-b of –0.26 and –0.32 for the US and Canada, respectively), rather than the evaluation of care received in the past (tau-b of –0.18 for both countries), seem to be more influential in the desire for health care system reform. Our data also show that satisfaction with one's insurance plan depresses the willingness to ask for reforms in the US in a significant fashion (tau-b of –0.22).

Support for reform is also related to political attitudes. We have previously suggested that political attitudes probably play a more important role in the US than in Canada due to the recent polarization of the debate over health care south of the border. The data from Table 7.2 seem to confirm this hypothesis.

Table 7.2 Opinion about the Role of Government and Support for Health Care Reform in Canada and the US

Canada				
Role for Government	***Minor Changes***	***Major Changes***	***Completely Rebuilt***	**%**
1 (person on his own)	37	48	14	9
2	38	52	10	13
3	43	51	6	45
4	44	49	7	18
5 (government sees)	35	53	11	14
US				
Role for Government	***Minor Canges***	***Major Changes***	***Completely Rebuilt***	**%**
1 (person on his own)	43	40	17	16
2	35	53	12	17
3	25	56	18	40
4	22	55	23	16
5 (government sees)	16	38	46	11

Notes: Sample sizes are 3,522 and 3,542 for Canada and the US, respectively (DKs are excluded). Data are weighted.

CANADA: $\chi 2 = 37.62$, $p < 0.000$ with 8 df; Cramer's V = 0.07; Kendall's Tau-B = –0.01, $p < 0.683$.

USA: $\chi 2 = 265$, $p < 0.000$ with 8 df; Cramer's V = 0.20; Kendall's Tau-B = 0.19, $p < 0.000$.

Question Wording: *"Role for Government" Variable:* Some people say that that the government in Ottawa (Washington) should see to it that every person has a job and a good standard of living. Other people say that the government should just let each person gets ahead on his own. And, of course, other people have opinions somewhere in between. Where would you place yourself on this scale, or haven't you thought much about this? (Variable recoded from 5 to 1). Percentages under the column % represent the proportion of the sample in each category for the "role for government" variable. Other entries represent the percentages of respondents supporting health care reform for each level of the role of government variable.

Respondents' views about the role of the state are linked quite closely to support for health care reform in the US, with the most interventionist respondents being more favorable to reform (tau-b of 0.19). However, this variable does not seem to exert any influence on support for reform in Canada (tau-b of –0.01).

One of the most central aspects of the debate over health care reform in the US has pitted those who believe that individuals must take steps to ensure that they have good health coverage against those who think that government has an important role to play in ensuring availability for all citizens. The same debate has also opposed those who believe that universal coverage either provided or regulated by the state is too expensive against those who believe the opposite. Canada, unlike the US, has not had such debates in recent times. Moreover, the issue of universal access to health care and coverage is the subject of a broad consensus in Canada, unlike in the US, where Republicans and Democrats disagree on this issue. The more recent and polarized debate over health care coverage in the US should ensure that the views on this issue are more closely related to support for health care system reform in the US than in Canada.

This hypothesis seems to be confirmed by the results presented in Table 7.3. The relationship between respondents' views on the role of the state in the provision of health care and the cost of universal health care are much more closely related to support for reform in the US (tau-b of 0.29

Table 7.3 Attitudes toward Health Care and Support for Health Care Reform in Canada and the US

Panel A. Health Insurance Plan

Canada				
Health Insurance Plan	***Minor Changes***	***Major Changes***	***Completely Rebuilt***	**%**
1 (individuals)	33	34	33	3
2	36	48	16	4
3	37	56	7	35
4	46	49	5	24
5 (government)	43	49	8	35
US				
Health Insurance Plan	***Minor Changes***	***Major Changes***	***Completely Rebuilt***	**%**
1 (individuals)	51	35	13	13
2	43	49	8	13
3	29	56	16	37
4	17	62	21	16
5 (government)	14	44	42	22

(Continued)

Table 7.3 (Continued)

Panel B. Universality

	Canada			
Universality	*Minor Changes*	*Major Changes*	*Completely Rebuilt*	%
1 (too costly)	26	48	26	6
2	34	58	9	6
3	40	53	8	30
4	45	51	5	19
5 (do everything)	43	49	8	40
	US			
Universality	*Minor Changes*	*Major Changes*	*Completely Rebuilt*	%
1 (too costly)	44	40	16	18
2	39	51	11	13
3	31	53	16	33
4	20	64	17	15
5 (do everything)	10	47	43	21

Notes: Sample sizes are 3,522 and 3,542 for Canada and the US, respectively (DKs are excluded). Data are weighted.

Panel A: CANADA: $\chi2$ = 104.44, p < 0.000 with 8 df; Cramer's V = 0.12; Kendall's Tau-B = –0.06, p < 0.000.

Panel A: USA: $\chi2$ = 458.26, p < 0.000 with 8 df; Cramer's V = 0.26; Kendall's Tau-B = 0.29, p < 0.000.

Panel B: CANADA: $\chi2$ = 105.76, p < 0.000 with 8 df; Cramer's V = 0.12; Kendall's Tau-B = –0.08, p 0<.000.

Panel B: USA: $\chi2$ = 420.46, p < 0.000 with 8 df; Cramer's V = 0.25; Kendall's Tau-B = 0.26, p < 0.000.

Question Wording: *"Health Insurance Plan" Variable:* Some people say that that there should be a government insurance plan which would cover all medical and hospital expenses for everyone. Other people say that all medical expenses should be paid by individuals, and through private insurance plans like Blue Cross and other company-paid plans. And, of course, other people have opinions somewhere in between. Where would you place yourself on this scale, or haven't you thought much about this? (Reverse coding in table). *"Universality" Variable:* Some people say that ensuring that health care is universally available to everyone, regardless of their ability to pay, is so important that we must do everything to protect these principles. Other people say that ensuring universal access, regardless of ability to pay, is simply too costly and we cannot afford to expect so much from health care system. And, of course, other people have opinions somewhere in between. Where would you place yourself on this scale, or haven't you thought much about this? (Reverse coding in table). Percentages under the column % represent the proportion of the sample in each category for the "insurance" and "universality" variables. Other entries represent the percentages of respondents supporting health care reform for each level of "insurance" and "universality" variables.

and 0.26, respectively) than in Canada (tau-b of –0.06 and –0.08, respectively). Another very interesting piece of information is that the direction of association between these variables and demand for change differs from one country to the other. The negative relationship observed in Canada underlines once again that support for the idea of health care reform is associated with a withdrawal of the state in favor of the private sector. The positive relationship in the American case shows instead that the concept of health care reform means a greater role for the state for most citizens. The results presented here therefore appear logical to the extent that "reform" signifies a break with the present situation. For Canadians, this means a very large role for the state in the health policy sector, and for Americans, the reverse. With this in mind, "reform" is therefore synonymous with privatization in Canada and increased state intervention in the US. Given the differences in the nature and intensity of debates in both countries, it is not surprising that a generally favorable attitude toward the state, and its involvement in health care in particular, is strongly and positively related to the demand for change in the US and weakly and negatively related to support for reform in Canada.

In Canada, opinions about the health care system are less likely to be related to support for health care reform except for the question of the symbolic value of the health system in defining Canadian identity. As shown in Table 7.4,

Table 7.4 Opinion about Perceptions of the Health System as Unifying Symbol and Support for Health Care Reform in Canada and the US

		Canada		
Unifying Symbol	***Minor Changes***	***Major Changes***	***Completely Rebuilt***	**%**
No	29	59	12	32
Yes	46	47	7	69
		US		
Unifying Symbol	***Minor Changes***	***Major Changes***	***Completely Rebuilt***	**%**
No	26	52	22	73
Yes	31	49	20	27

Notes: Sample sizes are 3,522 and 3,542 for Canada and the US, respectively (DKs are excluded). Data are weighted.

CANADA: $\chi 2 = 99.18$, $p < 0.000$ with 2 df; Cramer's V = 0.17; Kendall's Tau-B = –0.17, $p < 0.000$.

USA: $\chi 2 = 6.02$, $p < 0.05$ with 2 df; Cramer's V = 0.04; Kendall's Tau-B = –0.04, $p < 0.025$.

Question Wording: *"Symbol" Variable:* Do you consider the health service system as a unifying symbol of your country and its people? Percentages under the column % represent the proportion of the sample in each category for the "symbol" variable. Other entries represent the percentages of respondents supporting health care reform for respondents answering "no" or "yes" to this question.

while nearly seven Canadians out of ten (69%) agree with the statement that the health care system of their country is an important component of their national identity, only 27% of Americans feel the same in terms of their own country. Moreover, the link between this opinion and support for health care reform is much stronger in Canada than in the US (tau-b of –0.17 and –0.04, respectively). As expected, Canadians who give symbolic value to their own health care system are also those who are the most reluctant to see it change.

Sociotropic perceptions can also influence support for reform. A person who believes that the quality of health care has generally improved in recent years may be less inclined to think that changes are necessary. The data in Table 7.5 confirm this expectation and show the strength of the relationship

Table 7.5 Assessments of Evolution of Health Care and Support for Health Care Reforms in Canada and the US

Canada				
Evolution of Health Care	***Minor Changes***	***Major Changes***	***Completely Rebuilt***	**%**
1 (greatly deteriorated)	4	60	36	6
2	20	69	11	24
3 (stayed the same)	48	47	5	57
4	66	30	4	11
5 (greatly improved)	63	24	13	1
US				
Evolution of Health Care	***Minor Changes***	***Major Changes***	***Completely Rebuilt***	**%**
1 (greatly deteriorated)	4	29	67	6
2	13	60	27	24
3 (stayed the same)	31	53	16	51
4	47	43	10	16
5 (greatly improved)	62	19	20	3

Notes: Sample sizes are 3,522 and 3,542 for Canada and the US, respectively (DKs are excluded). Data are weighted.

CANADA: $\chi2$ = 566.34, $p < 0.000$ with 8 df; Cramer's V = 0.29; Kendall's Tau-B = –0.33, $p < 0.000$.

USA: $\chi2$ = 561.60, $p < 0.000$ with 8 df; Cramer's V = 0.29; Kendall's Tau-B = –0.31, $p < 0.000$.

Question Wording: *"Evolution of Health Care" Variable:* In your opinion, has the quality of health care in your country over the past two years deteriorated, improved or stayed the same? Please respond using a 5-point scale where 1 means greatly deteriorated, 5 means greatly improved, the mid-point 3 means stayed the same. Percentages under the column % represent the proportion of the sample in each category for the "evolution of health care" variable. Other entries represent the percentages of respondents supporting health care reform for each level of assessment of the "evolution of health care" variable.

between these sociotropic and retrospective perceptions (the survey question in this case asks the respondent to determine whether the quality of care has improved, deteriorated, or stayed the same over the past two years) in both Canada and the US (tau-b of –0.33 and –0.31, respectively).

This section has made use of bivariate analysis to describe the determinants of support for health care system reform in the US and Canada. The next section focuses on a more complete model and will discuss multivariate analyses that will better assess the specific contribution of the factors mentioned above.

A MODEL OF DEMAND FOR REFORMS IN THE US AND CANADA

We will now discuss a comprehensive model of support for health care system reform in the US and Canada using the same approach as in the previous two chapters—that is, by using blocks of variables that are successively introduced into the analysis in order to test their impact on the dependent variable. The model that will be used in both countries will examine in stages the impact of the different types of variables analyzed in the previous chapters (socioeconomic characteristics, egotropic perceptions, ideological and political attitudes, opinions on health care systems, sociotropic perceptions) to which we will add a sixth block of variables including respondents' opinions about the health care system in their own country and in the neighboring country (US for Canadians and vice versa; see Chapter 6 for a detailed discussion about these new variables). Estimation remains via ordered logistic regression since our dependent variable in this chapter is still ordinal in nature, like our two previous ones.

Findings about the determinants of an individual's desire for change to their own health care system are presented in Tables 7.6 and 7.7. A first striking result is the weak effect of socio-demographic variables in explaining support for health care system reform. Nonetheless, two results stand out: the variables of age and living in Quebec. The elderly, more in contact with the health system and more concerned about the quality of care, show a greater willingness to see reform come about in their respective countries (this result emerges in the more elaborated models for the US; see Table 7.6, columns 2 to 6). The case of Quebec was discussed in the previous section and the multivariate analysis highlights the major impact (the coefficient is 1.42 in the model of column 1, Table 7.6) and resilience of this variable. The "Quebec" variable, similar to the "age" variable, is still statistically significant in the full model that includes 28 variables and even keeps close to three-fourths of its original effect (see last column of Table 7.6).

The second model, which includes egotropic perceptions, underlines the importance of these variables; when these variables are introduced, the pseudo R^2 increases from 0.10 to 0.26 and from 0.00 to 0.15 in the

Table 7.6 Determinants of Support for Reforms of the Canadian Health Care System

DV: Reforms(CAN)	Model 1	Model 2	Model 3	Model 4	Model 5	Model 6
AB	0.41**	0.25	0.22	0.23	0.16	0.14
	(0.13)	(0.15)	(0.15)	(0.15)	(0.15)	(0.16)
BC	0.13	−0.07	−0.06	−0.05	−0.01	−0.19
	(0.12)	(0.13)	(0.14)	(0.14)	(0.14)	(0.15)
QC	1.42***	1.42***	1.32***	1.23***	1.25***	1.06***
	(0.10)	(0.12)	(0.13)	(0.13)	(0.14)	(0.15)
Atlantic	−0.19	−0.21	−0.19	−0.17	−0.06	−0.14
	(0.15)	(0.17)	(0.17)	(0.17)	(0.18)	(0.19)
Prairies	−0.22	0.00	0.02	−0.01	0.18	0.22
	(0.16)	(0.18)	(0.18)	(0.19)	(0.19)	(0.20)
Male	−0.02	0.15	0.13	0.17	0.19*	0.08
	(0.08)	(0.09)	(0.09)	(0.09)	(0.09)	(0.10)
Age	0.01***	0.01**	0.01*	0.01**	0.01**	0.01**
	(0.00)	(0.00)	(0.00)	(0.00)	(0.00)	(0.00)
Education	−0.01	0.00	0.01	0.01	0.01	0.01
	(0.02)	(0.03)	(0.03)	(0.03)	(0.03)	(0.03)
Gvt. emp.	−0.04	0.06	0.03	0.02	0.01	0.13
	(0.12)	(0.13)	(0.13)	(0.13)	(0.13)	(0.14)
Income	−0.01	0.02	0.01	0.02	0.02	0.03
	(0.01)	(0.01)	(0.01)	(0.01)	(0.01)	(0.02)
Past2years: egotropic (high)		−0.87*** (0.21)	−0.85*** (0.21)	−0.64** (0.21)	−0.26 (0.22)	0.14 (0.25)
Risk scale (high)		3.14***	3.21***	3.27***	2.80***	2.50***
		(0.20)	(0.20)	(0.20)	(0.21)	(0.23)
CANnopid			−0.07	−0.10	−0.14	−0.07
			(0.13)	(0.13)	(0.13)	(0.14)
Liberal			−0.22	−0.13	−0.16	−0.08
			(0.12)	(0.12)	(0.13)	(0.13)
NDP			0.05	0.12	0.01	0.11
			(0.15)	(0.16)	(0.16)	(0.17)
Bloc			0.40*	0.39	0.27	0.23
			(0.20)	(0.20)	(0.21)	(0.23)
Green			0.66	0.80	0.88*	0.82
			(0.42)	(0.42)	(0.44)	(0.45)

DV: Reforms(CAN)	Model 1	Model 2	Model 3	Model 4	Model 5	Model 6
Ideology (right)			0.88***	0.77***	0.90***	0.72**
			(0.23)	(0.24)	(0.24)	(0.26)
Government role (more)			–0.45*	–0.33	–0.23	–0.23
			(0.18)	(0.18)	(0.19)	(0.20)
Individualism scale (more)			–0.42	–0.83**	–0.83**	–0.74**
			(0.25)	(0.26)	(0.27)	(0.28)
Gov. insurance plan				–0.05	–0.05	0.00
				(0.05)	(0.06)	(0.06)
Universal access				–0.26	–0.23	–0.11
				(0.19)	(0.19)	(0.22)
Public system: symbol				–0.26*	–0.32*	–0.28*
				(0.12)	(0.13)	(0.14)
Health care system: symbol				–0.50***	–0.49***	–0.35**
				(0.11)	(0.11)	(0.12)
Past2years: sociotropic (high)					–2.97***	–2.35***
					(0.26)	(0.28)
Opinion about own HCS(CAN)						–2.04***
						(0.26)
Opinion about neighbor HCS(CAN)						0.70***
						(0.20)
Cut 1 (constant)	0.22	1.31***	1.29***	0.51	–0.71	–1.12*
	(0.19)	(0.28)	(0.37)	(0.40)	(0.43)	(0.47)
Cut 2 (constant)	3.17***	4.60***	4.62***	3.90***	2.86***	2.49***
	(0.20)	(0.30)	(0.39)	(0.41)	(0.43)	(0.47)
N	2,817	2,424	2,424	2,424	2,388	2,112
Pseudo R^2	0.10	0.26	0.27	0.29	0.34	0.37

Notes: Data are weighted. Entries are ordered logistic regression coefficients with standard errors in parentheses. Pseudo R^2 are Nagelkerke. $^{*}p < 0.05$, $^{**}p < 0.01$, $^{***}p < 0.001$. For the description of the variables, see the Appendix.

Canadian and US models, respectively. Further interesting findings stand out from this second block of variables. First, it may be noted that support for reform is more related to the quality of care that respondents expect to receive in the future than the quality of care that they have received in the past. The coefficients that tap into prospective perceptions, measuring the

Table 7.7 Determinants of Reforms of the US Health Care System

DV: Reforms(USA)	Model 1	Model 2	Model 3	Model 4	Model 5	Model 6
South	0.12	0.10	0.16	0.15	0.16	0.21*
	(0.07)	(0.08)	(0.08)	(0.08)	(0.09)	(0.10)
Male	–0.13*	–0.02	–0.00	0.01	0.11	0.16
	(0.07)	(0.08)	(0.08)	(0.08)	(0.08)	(0.10)
Age	–0.00	0.01*	0.01***	0.01**	0.01	0.01**
	(0.00)	(0.00)	(0.00)	(0.00)	(0.00)	(0.00)
Education	0.02	0.05	0.02	0.01	0.02	0.03
	(0.02)	(0.03)	(0.03)	(0.03)	(0.03)	(0.04)
Black	–0.00	0.03	–0.27*	–0.22	–0.12	–0.22
	(0.10)	(0.12)	(0.13)	(0.13)	(0.14)	(0.16)
Gvt. emp.	–0.09	0.18	0.22	0.13	0.11	0.13
	(0.16)	(0.17)	(0.18)	(0.18)	(0.18)	(0.21)
Income	–0.02	0.02	0.03*	0.04**	0.04**	0.03
	(0.01)	(0.01)	(0.01)	(0.01)	(0.01)	(0.02)
SatINS		–0.72***	–0.61***	–0.51***	–0.31*	0.11
		(0.14)	(0.14)	(0.14)	(0.15)	(0.18)
Past2years:		–1.07***	–0.92***	–0.81***	–0.26	–0.31
egotropic (high)		(0.22)	(0.22)	(0.23)	(0.24)	(0.29)
Risk scale (high)		1.86***	1.75***	1.72***	1.44***	1.29***
		(0.15)	(0.16)	(0.16)	(0.17)	(0.20)
USAnopid			0.15	0.09	0.13	0.21
			(0.11)	(0.11)	(0.11)	(0.13)
Democrat			0.04	–0.02	0.06	0.09
			(0.12)	(0.13)	(0.13)	(0.15)

Ideology (conservative)			−0.62***	−0.27	−0.34	0.23
			(0.18)	(0.19)	(0.19)	(0.23)
Government role (more)			0.61***	0.21	0.22	0.40
			(0.16)	(0.18)	(0.18)	(0.21)
Individualism scale (more)			−1.22***	−0.65**	−0.64**	−0.31
			(0.21)	(0.23)	(0.23)	(0.28)
Gov. insurance plan				0.27***	0.26***	0.18**
				(0.05)	(0.05)	(0.06)
Universal access				0.54**	0.58***	0.48*
				(0.17)	(0.17)	(0.21)
Private system: symbol				−0.03	0.02	0.26*
				(0.09)	(0.09)	(0.11)
Health care system: symbol				−0.30***	−0.16	−0.08
				(0.09)	(0.10)	(0.11)
Past2years: sociotropic (high)					−2.68***	−1.89***
					(0.22)	(0.26)
Opinion about own HCS (USA)						−2.45***
						(0.22)
Opinion about neighbor HCS(USA)						0.89***
						(0.22)
Cut 1 (constant)	−1.03***	−0.53*	−0.96**	0.01	−0.81*	−0.32
	(0.18)	(0.27)	(0.35)	(0.36)	(0.38)	(0.47)
Cut 2 (constant)	1.22***	2.02***	1.72***	2.77***	2.08***	2.80***
	(0.18)	(0.27)	(0.35)	(0.37)	(0.38)	(0.47)
N	3,164	2,476	2,476	2,476	2,438	1,807
Pseudo R^2	0.004	0.15	0.22	0.25	0.31	0.39

Notes: Data are weighted. Entries are ordered logistic regression coefficients with standard errors in parentheses. Pseudo R^2 are Nagelkerke. $^{*}p < 0.05$, $^{**}p < 0.01$, $^{***}p < 0.001$. For the description of the variables, see the Appendix.

expected risk of no longer receiving quality care, are statistically significant in both countries, and their magnitude is larger than the indicator for quality of care received in the past (the coefficients in columns 2 of Tables 7.6 and 7.7 for the risk variable are 3.14 for Canada and 1.86 for the US, while the coefficients associated with the evaluation of past care are –0.87 and –1.07 for these two countries). A second result is worth noting. We have earlier stipulated that the expected performance of the health system would play a greater role in Canada than in the US. The results confirm this intuition. The size of the coefficient linked to the risk of no longer receiving quality care in the future is significantly higher in Canada (3.14) than in the US (1.86). These results seem to confirm that the framing of the debate around universality, which has served Canadians well in the past, may no longer be viable in the near future, given the country's aging population and the soaring costs of health care accompanying this demographic change. In this context, reforms appear to be necessary. Fear of the future is therefore a significantly larger determinant of support for health care reform in Canada than in the US. Finally, and tellingly, a strong and significant relationship is observed between the perceived quality of one's insurance and the willingness to ask for reforms (–0.72). This confirms once again that respondents who are satisfied with their current coverage are more inclined to stick with the status quo than ask for reforms in the US.

The debate over health care is much more politically and ideologically polarized in the US than it is in Canada. We should therefore expect that views on health care reform reflect this polarization more in the former than in the latter. The results of the regression analyses (see column 3 of Tables 7.6 and 7.7) generally confirm this expectation. However, the first observation to be made is that partisan identification does not seem to have an important impact on either side of the border (the case of Bloc Québécois supporters, limited to the province of Quebec, is more a reflection of public opinion in this province than any real partisan polarization). That said, the overall effect of political attitudes (which include ideological self-positioning and opinions on the role of the state, as well as an individualism scale) is much higher in the US than in Canada: the three variables measuring these attitudes are significant in the US, but only two are in Canada. Furthermore, the pseudo R^2 values increase three percentage points when these variables are included in the former case and only one percentage point in the latter case. The results also confirm that supporters of reform come from different political backgrounds in both countries. In Canada, conservatives are the ones who demand reform whereas in the US it is liberals who support it (note the opposite signs of the variables for ideology and the role of government).

The intensity and recent nature of collective deliberation over an issue can help create a priming effect by making each side's arguments more salient. The debate over the health care system in Canada has become less intense in recent years (Soroka et al. 2013). The federal election of 2000 was the last election where different views about the health care system were at the heart of the campaign (Nadeau, Pétry, and Bélanger 2010; see also Chapter 2). The situation in the US is quite different. The debate over "Obamacare" has brought to the fore two clearly opposing conceptions of how the health system should function: one focused on individual responsibility and the other focused more on an active role for the government to ensure universality in access to health care.

The different paths that the health care debate has taken in Canada and the US, more distant and diffuse in the former and more recent and structured in the latter, suggest that views about the balance between individual and collective responsibilities in the functioning of the health system will be much more pervasive among Americans than Canadians. The results strongly confirm this hypothesis (see column 4 in Tables 7.6 and 7.7). While those who think the government should put in place an insurance plan providing universal health care (see variable "Gov. insurance plan") despite it being costly (see variable "Universal access") are more likely to support health care reform in the US (the coefficients are statistically significant in both cases and are 0.27 and 0.54), opinions on these issues contribute nothing in the Canadian case as to whether one is for or against health care reform (interestingly, the impact of the variable related to an individual's own health insurance is still negative and significant in this model).

We can therefore generally conclude that attitudes and ideological considerations weigh less heavily in the assessment of the health system and in supporting its possible reform in Canada as compared to the US. That said, one part of Canadians' views on their health care system seems to rest on ideological grounds, namely the idea that the current universal system in place is a uniquely Canadian feature that helps cement national unity. In short, in the eyes of many Canadians their health care system is a symbol, an opinion much less widespread in the US. This opinion, held with great conviction by some, constitutes an obstacle to any reform, as shown by the results in Tables 7.6 and 7.7 (column 4). It can be seen in the Canadian case that recognizing the health care system as a component of Canadian identity exerts a stronger influence (and negative as one would expect) on supporting change than in the US (the coefficients are –0.50 in the first case and –0.30 in the second). The negative sign of the variable in both cases is easily explained because in Canada it is the "public" nature of the system that is the hallmark, with the reverse being true in the US. Insofar as reform plans go against this characterization in both countries, it is not surprising that those who give symbolic value to the health system in the US and Canada may be less favorable to any idea of change.

Earlier, we examined the effect of egotropic perceptions on support for reform. Work on public opinion, especially on economic voting (see notably Nadeau, Lewis-Beck, and Bélanger 2013), has shown the strong impact of sociotropic perceptions on policy choices. The same logic applies in this case. A positive assessment of recent developments in the quality of health care should reduce the desire for reform, with the reverse being true in the case of a negative assessment. The results (see column 5 in Tables 7.6 and 7.7) indicate that this variable has a significant impact in both Canada and the US: the coefficients that are associated with these attitudes are –2.97 and –2.68, respectively, and the inclusion of these variables into the model contributes by itself to a rise of three percentage points in terms of the variation explained in both cases.

An interesting aspect of the health care debates in both Canada and the US is that the situation in the adjacent country plays a significant role in collective deliberation over the national health system (see Marmor 1993; Nadeau et al. 2010). The situation in Canada will be used either as a model by advocates of reform in the US or as a foil by those who oppose it. The situation in the US will similarly be exploited and demonized by opponents of increased privatization in the Canadian system, while supporters of a change of this nature will invoke the effectiveness of the American system and shorter waiting times for treatment.

An even more remarkable aspect of these US-Canada dynamics is that they are not limited to specialists and members of pressure groups. The data in the previous chapter showed the consistency of these cross-border opinions. What remains to be determined is whether these consistent opinions on both sides of the border have a significant impact on support for reform. In this case, the expectation is clear. Given the very different nature of health systems in the two countries, a favorable opinion of the American system should have a positive effect on support for changes to Canada (going toward American-style privatization), while for Americans, a favorable opinion would mean sympathy toward a more "socialist" system like that of Canada. The innovative nature of this hypothesis requires that it be tested with all possible precautions. This is why two variables are introduced into the equations to estimate the latter model. First, as it should be, there is a variable measuring the views of Canadians toward the American system and vice versa. Also included for both countries is a question that has the same wording ("What is your overall feeling of the health care system?") but toward one's own national health system rather than that of the neighboring country.

The results for the final model that estimates support for health care reform are presented in column 6 of Tables 7.6 and 7.7. Out of more than two dozen variables in the models, the list of statistically significant variables is particularly interesting, which includes variables for Quebec, age, egotropic and prospective perceptions (note the stronger effect for the Canadian model), symbolism in Canada, opinions on universality in the US, and evaluations of recent performance of the health system. Our focus here is specifically on the impact of cross-border perceptions. To avoid overstating the effect of these perceptions, we introduced into the equation variables that measured respondents' overall perception of the health care system in their own country. As expected, these variables are strongly related to opinions on the desirability of reform. The large and negative coefficients associated with these variables, –2.04 in Canada and –2.45 in the US, confirm our expectation that support for reform decreases markedly among those who have an overall favorable impression of their own system health.

This last result is convincing, but not very surprising. That said, while the idea that Americans' and Canadians' perceptions of the health system of their neighboring country can influence their desires for change has been suggested, it has never been formally tested. And the results are clear. Canadians' perceptions about the US health care system and Americans' perceptions about the Canadian health care system significantly influence support for health care reform in these two countries. A Canadian's favorable opinion of the US health care system increases the likelihood that they will be in favor of reforming the Canadian health care system and vice versa. The coefficients related to cross-border perceptions are in line with what was postulated earlier, that is, positive and unequivocally statistically significant. The sheer size of these coefficients, 0.70 in Canada and 0.89 in the US, shows the importance of these effects, observed in the context of well-elaborated and complete multivariate models. This result seems to confirm that cross-border perceptions about the health care systems in North America are not only "real" but also that that they matter.

So far, the discussion about our results has been based on logistic regression coefficients. The changes in probabilities displayed in Tables 7.8 and 7.9 confirm all these findings. A few results are worth noticing. First, it is interesting to observe that fears about not being able to get required health care in the future (coefficient of 0.15 for the "risk" variable in column 6 of Table 7.8) is as important in Canada as "heavy" considerations such as overall judgments about the health care system (coefficient of –0.13) and assessments about the recent evolution of its quality (coefficient of –0.15). Second, it appears that prospective considerations also play a major role in the US in fuelling citizens' willingness for reform, the change in probability associated with the "risk" variable being roughly on par (0.16; see column 6 in Table 7.9) with the one observed in Canada. This finding nuances our previous conclusion about the higher impact of this variable in Canada and underlines the importance of prospective considerations in the formation of individuals' opinion about reforms in general. That said, the change in probability for the "risk" variable remains *relatively* higher in Canada compared to other "heavy" considerations (0.15versus –0.15 and –0.13) than is the case in the US (0.16 versus –0.24 and –0.31). A third finding stands out. The results suggest that opinions about the Canadian health care system matter more (0.11) in the debate about reforming the US system than the opposite (0.04). This result is likely due to the more recent and ongoing nature of the debate about the reform of the American health care system which may have contributed to priming the comparison with the Canadian system. One conjecture is that the opposite result could have been true at

Table 7.8 Change in Probabilities Related to Support for Reforms of the Canadian Health Care System

DV: Reforms(CAN)	Model 1	Model 2	Model 3	Model 4	Model 5	Model 6
AB	0.03	0.02	0.01	0.02	0.01	0.01
BC	0.01	–0.00	–0.00	–0.00	–0.00	–0.01
QC	0.11	0.10	0.09	0.08	0.08	0.07
Atlantic	–0.01	–0.01	–0.01	–0.01	–0.00	–0.01
Prairies	–0.02	0.00	–0.00	–0.00	0.01	0.01
Male	–0.00	0.01	0.01	0.01	0.01	0.01
Age	0.001	0.001	0.000	0.001	0.000	0.001
Education	–0.00	0.00	0.00	0.00	0.00	0.00
Gvt. emp.	–0.00	0.00	0.00	0.00	0.00	0.01
Income	–0.000	0.001	0.001	0.001	0.001	0.002
Past 2 years: egotropic (high)		–0.06	–0.06	–0.04	–0.02	0.01
Risk scale (high)		0.22	0.22	0.22	0.18	0.15
CANnopid			–0.00	–0.01	–0.01	–0.00
Liberal			–0.02	–0.01	–0.01	–0.01
NDP			0.00	0.01	0.00	0.01
Bloc			0.03	0.03	0.02	0.01
Green			0.05	0.05	0.06	0.05
Ideology (right)			0.06	0.05	0.06	0.04
Government role (more)			–0.03	–0.02	–0.01	–0.01
Individualism scale (more)			–0.03	–0.06	–0.05	–0.05
Gov. insurance plan				–0.00	–0.00	0.00
Universal access				–0.02	–0.01	–0.01
Public system: symbol				–0.02	–0.02	–0.02
Health care system: symbol				–0.03	–0.03	–0.02
Past 2 years: sociotropic (high)					–0.19	–0.15
Opinion about own HCS(CAN)						–0.13
Opinion about neighbor HCS(CAN)						0.04

Notes: Entries in the table are the changes in probability that the dependent variable takes its highest value (completely rebuilt) when an explanatory variable varies from its minimum to its maximum value. All calculations were performed with Stata 11.0.

Table 7.9 Change in Probabilities Related to Support for Reforms of the US Health Care System

DV: Reforms(USA)	Model 1	Model 2	Model 3	Model 4	Model 5	Model 6
South	0.02	0.01	0.02	0.02	0.02	0.02
Male	–0.02	–0.00	–0.00	0.00	0.01	0.02
Age	–0.000	0.001	0.001	0.001	0.001	0.001
Education	0.00	0.01	0.00	0.00	0.00	0.00
Black	–0.00	0.01	–0.04	–0.03	–0.02	–0.03
Gvt. emp.	–0.01	0.03	0.03	0.02	0.01	0.02
Income	–0.003	0.002	0.005	0.005	0.005	0.003
SatINS		–0.11	–0.09	–0.07	–0.04	0.01
Past 2 years: egotropic (high)		–0.16	–0.13	–0.11	–0.03	–0.04
Risk scale (high)		0.28	0.25	0.24	0.19	0.16
USAnopid			0.02	0.01	0.02	0.03
Democrat			0.01	–0.00	0.01	0.01
Ideology (conservative)			–0.09	–0.04	–0.04	0.03
Government role (more)			0.09	0.03	0.03	0.05
Individualism scale (more)			–0.17	–0.09	–0.09	–0.04
Gov. insurance plan				0.04	0.03	0.03
Universal access				0.08	0.08	0.06
Private system: symbol				–0.00	0.00	0.03
Health care system: symbol				–0.04	–0.02	–0.01
Past2years: sociotropic (high)					–0.35	–0.24
Opinion about own HCS (USA)						–0.31
Opinion about neighbor HCS(USA)						0.11

Notes: Entries in the table are the changes in probability that the dependent variable takes its highest value (completely rebuilt) when an explanatory variable varies from its minimum to its maximum value. All calculations were performed with Stata 11.0.

the time of the 2000 Canadian federal election, which was fought to a large extent on the opportunity to transform the national health care system into a type of American, two-tier kind of system (see Chapter 2). The major conçlusion remains, however. Assessments about the neighbor's health care system matter in the formation of Americans' and Canadians' opinion about the opportunity to reform their own health care system.

CONCLUSION

The overall goal of our study on the opinions and perceptions of Americans and Canadians about various aspects of their own health care system was to see if their overall judgment was positive and what motivated some to press for reforms. From our study, three observations emerge. First, Americans are generally less satisfied with their health care system than Canadians and are more likely to demand significant health system reform. Second, public opinion in both countries on the desirability of health care reform has changed over the past twenty-five years. While Canadians were reluctant to reform their health care system in the late 1980s, they expressed strong dissatisfaction about its operation during the 1990s before returning to a less severe judgment of it in recent years. In the US, the trajectory of public opinion was different. The dissatisfaction of Americans toward their health care system, along with their desire to see reform, has been constant for a quarter century before taking a change for the positive in the wake of the debate over "Obamacare." Thus, we have witnessed over time a convergence of Canadian and US public opinion where support for reform is concerned. A quarter century ago, the contrast was striking between Canadians' satisfaction with their own health care system and Americans' deep dissatisfaction with their respective health care system. Today, things have changed, and while citizens of both countries express moderate dissatisfaction, it is still more prominent in the US. Third, our study on support for reform should be put into perspective. In the Canadian case, the debate over health care was less intense at the time of the survey (spring 2011) and revolved around the desirability of increasing the private sector's role in the delivery of health care in Canada. In the American case, the debate raged on over the appropriateness of adopting a binding legislative framework that would ensure better coverage for all Americans, especially those without health insurance.

The debate over health care reform means different things in both countries. In Canada, reform means "less government," and in the US it means "more government." The results of our analyses must be interpreted in this light, as a brief review of the main findings will clearly show. The desire for reform peaks in the province of Quebec, where dissatisfaction with the health care system is deep. The results also highlight the similarities and differences about the determinants of support for reform in both countries. The most notable differences deal with the ideological profile of those who support change. In Canada, change is supported by segments of the population who are more conservative and hostile to government intervention, while the opposite is true in the US.

Another marked difference is the fact that the debate over health care in the US is more current, intense, and polarized than in Canada, which has contributed to making certain considerations stick out in the minds of Americans. Consequently, Americans' ideological predispositions (e.g., conservative versus liberal, the role of the state, individualism), as well as their specific views on the health care system (e.g., individual versus collective responsibility in ensuring health care coverage, the principle of universality) are much more related to support for reform in the US than in Canada. This result confirms once again that the issue of health care is much more of a positional issue in the US and a valence issue in Canada. This valence dimension in Canada combines with Canadians' strong disposition to see their own health system as part of their collective identity. Nearly three out of four Canadians believe that their health care system is a unifying symbol of identity; similar views are shared by only one in four Americans regarding their own system. The pervasiveness of this belief in Canada limits the possibility of change but also probably explains the consensual nature of Canadian opinion about the main principles guiding the operation of the health system. In this context, the debates in Canada focus more on the managerial capacity of governments to effectively operate a system based on generally accepted principles rather than on the principles themselves.

Despite the differences, there are also similarities in the determinants of support for reform in the two countries. The elderly, those who believe that the quality of care has deteriorated, those who are not satisfied with their health insurance plan in the US, those who are unhappy with the care that they have received in the past, and those who are concerned about health care that they will receive in the future express a clear desire for change in both Canada and the US. That said, one difference emerges among these similarities. The desire for change in Canada seems to be less driven by dissatisfaction with the care received in the past than concerns about the quality of the care that they will receive in the future. Canadians seem to believe that the universal basis of their health care system produced good results in the past, but that this principle may be unsustainable in the future. This mixture of satisfaction with the past and pessimism about the future is much more decisive in determining support for change in Canada than it is in the US.

A final result worth noting focuses on the impact of cross-border perceptions on support for health care system reform. It is not unusual to see public policy experts' opinions be influenced by practices in other countries. It is also arguably something that can occur among those leading public opinion as well as among groups particularly interested in a certain issue. What seems remarkable in this case is the fact that large segments of the Canadian and US population had a well-defined opinion of the health system in operation in their neighboring country. Even more remarkable is the fact that these opinions had a significant impact on the debate and support for health reform in both countries. A favorable image of the US health care system is positively related to support for reform in Canada, with the same thing being true about the debate in the US; Americans with a favorable opinion of the Canadian system are those who are quick to support the idea of changing the health care system in their country.

This result is all the more remarkable given that the word "reform," as discussed previously, has different meanings in the US and Canada. This means that the profile of individuals who have a positive image of the health system of their neighboring country will also be different; this was confirmed by the analysis in the previous chapter. In short, the most conservative people in Canada appreciate the American system the most, and their positive assessment of it confirms their opinion about the need to give a greater role to the private sector in the provision of health care in Canada. Conversely, the most liberal people in the US like the Canadian system because of its collective orientation, and their positive image of it reinforces their commitment to reforms in their own country.

Conclusion

Health care policy is a central concern for citizens of advanced democracies. Our understanding of the determinants of individuals' opinions on this important policy issue has been both limited and scattered, however. This study has tried to add to our knowledge of this topic by making use of a unique comparative body of survey data from both the United States and Canada.

We discuss what we regard as our *most* significant findings below. That our findings are important for those interested in health care policy is, we hope, relatively clear. But we also want to make clear that we regard the preceding chapters as contributing not just to what we know about health care attitudes but also to public attitudes about policy more generally. We see this as an important addition to the broader literature focused on how (and indeed whether) citizens in modern democracies form their opinions about major public policy domains. Individuals' views about other issues, most notably the economy (see Lewis-Beck and Stegmaier 2007), have been studied extensively. We now have a relatively good sense not just for where attitudes about the economy come from but also how these attitudes matter to policy preferences and government support. The same cannot (yet) be said about health care policy. With this work in hand, however, we hope to be one step further along in this regard.

Indeed, one general conclusion to be drawn from our results concerns respondents' high level of sophistication in their evaluations of health care–related issues. The multifaceted nature of these evaluations—egotropic, sociotropic, retrospective, and prospective—underlines citizens' well-grounded and elaborated opinions about their health care system. Just as past work has found structure to public attitudes on the economy or on foreign policy, we have found structure to public attitudes on health care. This is of real significance.

Moreover, our findings make clear that exploring the mix of retrospective and prospective considerations that individuals bring to bear matters for our understanding of health care policy attitudes—when they assess the current performance of their health care system, and when they contemplate the opportunity to reform it. Results from Chapter 5 clearly show that citizens' current levels of satisfaction toward the quality and delivery of health care in their country is, from an individual point of view (egotropic perceptions), tightly linked to assessments of its past *and* (expected) future performance. Results from Chapter 7 underline that the dominant egotropic motivation for reform is, in contrast, the anticipated performance of the system in the future. The interplay between the level of satisfaction with the present and the degree of optimism about the future plays a central role in the formation of Americans' and Canadians' opinions toward their health care system. We tend to believe that similar dynamics are at work in the formation of public opinion on many other policy issues.

Our focus has been on cross-sectional, individual-level survey data, but our findings provide some of the micro-level bases for what others have seen in aggregate-level trends in public opinion. Longitudinal work on health care policy in the US and Canada makes clear that publics both react to, and drive, public policymaking (see, for example, Soroka and Wlezien 2010). The preceding chapters reveal some of the sources of these aggregate-level shifts—they have explored some of the attitudes underlying the public opinion "signal" that can drive policy change.

The chapters mentioned here also make clear the degree to which public attitudes toward health care react to existing policies—consider the way in which the American public reacts to difficulties with access to a private system by increasingly supporting a public one, and the growing interest among Canadians, in reaction to access issues in a public system, in privatization. The detailed results presented in this book about the individual-level opinion formation process of Americans' and Canadians' views on health care reinforce the notion that public opinion can be informed and rational (Page and Shapiro 1992; Bélanger and Pétry 2005), and thus (1) a valuable input to public policymaking and (2) a powerful incentive for politicians to represent public interests.

Our study points to other ways in which public opinion is conditioned by political context as well. Americans' and Canadians' attitudes regarding the performance criteria of health care systems seem to largely overlap. However, they are expressed in two fundamentally different contexts: one where the constituent principles of the health care system are based on consensus, and the other where citizens form two rather distinct ideological and partisan groups. The roots of these differences can be traced long into the past, as described in Chapter 2. Different forces, among them race and territory (see Boychuk 2008), and different interests made the health insurance systems in Canada and the US "part at the crossroads" (Maioni 1998) and evolve thereafter along divergent pathways.

These different historical trajectories have paved the way to the emergence of two systems organized around different views concerning the most efficient way to deliver health care and based on different ideas about whether accessibility to it should be universal and ensured through a publicly funded system or left to individuals' responsibility via a market-based system. These diverging evolutions, as we have argued in Chapter 2, form the backdrop of the present book in three ways.

First, they have created rather unique contexts in which to study the determinants of individuals' opinions about a major public policy domain. As neighboring countries having many things in common, the US and Canada have implemented two very different health care systems. The situation of these two countries is also notable in another way: it is a very rare case of where citizens in one country have well-defined opinions about the public policy of another country. A large number of Canadians have a strong opinion about the American health care system, and the opposite is true for a good number of Americans.

Second, the different evolutions of health care policy in the US and Canada have led to (and/or been a product of) very different debates about health care reform. Most notable given our data is the timing of those debates. Health was high on Canadians' political agenda in the 1990s and early 2000s. Citizens' dissatisfaction with the health care system, which peaked at that time, led to the creation of the Romanow Commission, whose mandate was to examine solutions aiming at improving the system's current performance and ensuring its sustainability in the future. Since then, things have been somewhat more subdued on the Canadian front. To the contrary, the election of Barack Obama in 2008 paved the way to an intense debate about the reform of the US health care system that still polarizes the American political forces and public opinion.

The timing of our fieldwork, at the height of the debate on Obamacare, has provided an opportune time to examine public opinion on health care. That said, the more recent and intense debate about the reform of the health care system in the US has made the various considerations surrounding this debate (public versus private, individual versus collective responsibility, efficiency versus fairness, etc.) more salient and thus more cognitively accessible to the US respondents (Zaller 1992). As the results reported in this book neatly show, these considerations play a more considerable role in opinions about health care—whether the satisfaction with one's own health care system (Chapter 5), the opinion about that of the neighboring country (Chapter 6), or the support for health care reforms (Chapter 7)—among our US sample than for our Canadian respondents. Issue salience may mean that US respondents have thought more about health care in the recent past, and thus formed more structured, sensible attitudes. But saliency is only one part of the explanation. Empirical evidence gathered when the debate about health care was at its height in Canada clearly shows that Canadians' attitudes on this issue never displayed the kind of intense partisan and ideological polarization typical of the American public opinion. Furthermore, a review of the reform agenda in Canada for the period 1990–2003 shows that truly significant changes in the health care system were simply off the radar screen (Chapter 2). We thus conclude that the observed differences between Americans' and Canadians' opinions about health care are solidly entrenched. It is quite possible of course that the immediacy of the debate about health care in the US at the time of our fieldwork has simply accentuated the polarization in the US and the differences between Americans' and Canadians' views on this issue. But this is largely a matter of degree, not of nature.

These observations are crucial for the central argument of this book. Acknowledging the important differences between Americans' and Canadians' opinions on health care should not obscure the many things they share in common. The data presented in the preceding chapters point to the fact that individuals' basic needs and expectations in both countries with regard to health care are, overall, quite similar. Individuals' opinions about health care across the borders are, as is the case for many other issues, performance-responsive. Furthermore, the differences in Americans' and Canadians' views about the role of the state are relatively minor. But when it comes to the best mix of public-private health care provision, Americans' and Canadians' views depart from each other.

The evidence presented in this book clearly suggests that the divergent orientations taken by the debates about health care in both countries—ideologically-oriented in the US and valence-oriented in Canada—go a long way toward explaining the marked differences between Americans' and Canadians' opinions regarding their health care system and that of their neighboring country. The framing of the debates on health care, characterized by the central role of partisanship in the US and by varying commitments to equality in access to care in both countries, has left a significant imprint on Americans' and Canadians' views about the principles and the organization that should govern a fair and efficient health care system.

The explanation for these cross-border differences reflects, in our view, both the demand side (individuals' needs and assessments) and supply side (partisan framing of the debate) of public opinion on health care. The differences in opinions across borders result from the interplay between these factors in the US and Canada. Despite similar needs and expectations about the performance of the health care system, Americans' and Canadians' different views about this question is mostly, but of course not solely, due to the way in which the debate about health care is framed in their respective country.

Third, the histories of health care in the US and Canada have led to very different perspectives on the necessary direction of future reforms. As noted, just as the US is moving closer to a public health care system, its northern neighbor—which already has such a system—is seeing increasing public consideration of a private system. As results in Chapter 7 underline, the target of reforms and the profile of reformers stand in sharp contrast from one country to the other. Calls for reforming the health care system in Canada come from the most conservative quarters among the population and advocate for a growing role for the private sector, the opposite being true for the US. The clarity of our findings concerning this contrast speaks to the well-grounded nature of citizens' opinion on health care across both sides of the border. It also raises the possibility that the two systems may eventually converge, a point to which we will return.

One central issue in the comparative study of public opinion is to establish if different groups of citizens use the same criteria and follow the same logic when they form their opinions about comparable political objects. In the case at hand, the question is the following: Do Americans and Canadians assess the performance of their health care system in the same way? The main conclusion to be drawn from the findings presented in Chapters 3 to 5 is a resounding no. Of course, direct experience with the system is a key determinant of respondents' level of satisfaction in both countries. Health problems represent a form of risk. Insurance is the best protection toward risk. In Canada, the insurance scheme for health problems is collective. In the US, it depends on individuals' socioeconomic characteristics (age, income, type of work, etc.). Not surprisingly, insurance and coverage are key components in the health care debate in the US, and much less so in Canada. Americans are mostly concerned with the accessibility and affordability of health care whereas Canadians' main quarrel with their health care system is wait times. These considerations strongly impact on respondents' overall evaluation of their personal experience at getting quality health care (Chapter 3), a key determinant in their global evaluation of the system (Chapter 5). Sociotropic considerations are also common to respondents from both countries. Those who believe that the overall quality of health care has improved (or at least remained the same) in the recent past are much more inclined to express a higher level of satisfaction toward the performance of the health care system.

That said, the key conclusion that emerges from the examination of the explanatory models of respondents' satisfaction toward the health care system is that Americans and Canadians use different schema while performing this evaluation. Canadians' assessments of their health care system basically tend to be performance-oriented, while their American counterparts' evaluations appear to be much more delivery-oriented. In other words, health care presents the basic characteristic of a valence issue in Canada and a positional issue in the US (see Chapter 5). In Canada, the foundations of the health care system are consensual to the point that they are perceived as forming a national symbol (see Chapter 4). The main object of debate in this case is the evaluation of the sitting governments (both federal and provincial) in their management of the system. In the US, by way of contrast, the heart of the debate concerns the foundations of the system and more precisely whether or not the government should play a larger role to ensure that all Americans benefit from an adequate coverage of their health care needs. The strong impact of "general" political attitudes, such as ideology (liberal versus conservative), opinions about the role of government (interventionism versus laissez-faire), and individualism on Americans' opinions about their own health care system and that of their neighboring country, compared to the absence of such relationships in the Canadian sample (see Chapters 4 to 7), neatly demonstrates that health care is fundamentally a valence issue in Canada and a positional issue in the US.

OPINIONS ABOUT HEALTH CARE: MASS LEVEL OR ELITE BASED?

We have assumed so far that the observed differences between American and Canadian mass opinions are "real," in the sense that they reflect genuine differences in citizens' preferences, perceptions, and opinions about the health care system. Attitudes about health care are well structured, certainly, and based in part on personal experience, as well as more general attitudes about the role of government. That said, we should consider the possibility that public attitudes are at least partly elite-driven.

This seems particularly relevant for cross-border perceptions (Chapter 6), since Americans and Canadians cannot possibly rely on their own personal experience to form judgments of the health care system of a neighboring country. Let us first consider these cross-border perceptions. We see three points as particularly telling. First, the results presented in Chapter 6 amply confirm the presumption about the uniqueness of the US-Canada comparison about health care. Not only do large proportions of respondents in both countries (more than 85% in Canada, 67% in the US) form cross-border perceptions, but they do so in a well-structured way. As expected, richer and more conservative Canadians hold a more positive opinion of the US health care system, the opposite being true for American respondents. Second, and more interestingly, these cross-border perceptions seem to be used in a coherent fashion by respondents when they evaluate the opportunity of reforming their own health care system. As the results in Chapter 7 show, holding a positive opinion of the American health care system increases the probability of supporting a greater role for the private sector in Canada; conversely, holding a positive view of the Canadian health care system increases the probability of backing the Obamacare reform which involves a larger role for the government in the operation of the system. The consistency of these findings is striking. Third, an examination of the models in Chapters 5 and 6 reveals that the same type of factors seem to impact respondents' opinions about their own health care system and that of the neighboring country.

In sum, just as there is a sensible structure to respondents' attitudes about their own health care system, there is a sensible structure to their attitudes about the system north or south of the border. Where do these attitudes come from? This question raises, for us at least, the possibility that attitudes are partly elite-driven.

A hasty reading of this book might lead the reader to conclude that differences in opinions with their health care systems are "explained" by distinct American and Canadian national mass opinions. A divided American mass opinion produces divided attitudes about satisfaction with the US health care system; a markedly less divided Canadian mass opinion causes more united attitudes regarding satisfaction with the Canadian health care system.

We suspect, however, that this "culturalist" unidirectional interpretation of the role of mass opinion understates the role of elite preferences and attitudes. Indeed, the evidence also supports an alternative interpretation emphasizing differences in the attitudes and preferences of American and Canadian governing elites toward their health care systems. These elite differences are in turn reflected by differences at the mass level. As we have seen in Chapter 2, Canadian governments did not pass compulsory health insurance in response to popular demand. Quite the contrary: the evidence is that government health insurance was implemented by the government in advance of mass opinion (Hacker 1998; Maioni 1998; Boychuk 2008).

Research on the "opinion-policy nexus" shows that government policies do not simply respond to the demands of the mass public. This is true in the US and in Canada (Mauser and Margolis 1992; Pétry and Mendelsohn 2004). There is an important and convincing literature in the US suggesting that health care policymaking has been at times fundamentally at odds with public preferences, that policy regularly reflects the interests of the wealthy and better organized, and that politicians in the US have been as likely to manipulate public attitudes as they have been to follow them (e.g., Jacobs and Shapiro 2000; Morone and Jacobs 2005).

These considerations raise a larger question: Do politicians tend to respond to public opinion? Past work suggests that they do, at least some if not much of the time, particularly in salient policy domains (see, for example, Soroka and Wlezien 2010). Indeed, as we have noted, there is evidence that in both the US and Canada health spending follows public preferences. So at least some of the attitudes that we examine in this book seem likely to structure policy development—not simply react to elite opinion. There is potential for elite leadership, clearly. But the opinion-policy nexus is bidirectional. Publics both follow and lead.

PARTISANSHIP AND HEALTH CARE POLICY

Parties and partisanship are critical factors in accounting for the differences in the evolution of, and current attitudes about, health care in the US and Canada. Parties are related to stories that focus on elite manipulation, on the undue influence of interest groups, and so on, certainly. But we highlight them in particular here because their impact is so readily evident in the preceding analyses of public opinion. In particular, we want to highlight the possibility that parties can contribute to a polarization of opinion, underpinned by partisan attachments. This dynamic is clear in the preceding analyses—it is one of the critical differences between the structure of attitudes on health care in the US and Canada.

Where Canada is concerned, in short, there are only very minor differences in health care attitudes across partisan groups. Conservatives are slightly more concerned about the system, and slightly more likely to consider private options. But the differences between Conservatives and Liberals, and even Conservatives and NDP supporters, are slight. This is in stark contrast to the US, where there is a powerful connection between partisanship and health care preferences.

What are the consequences of these partisan differences? Our view is that partisanship gets in the way of rational health care policy preferences. Just as partisan debate has been seen to constrain the development of health care policy in the US (see Chapter 2), partisan attachment unduly colors citizens' views of health care policy. This is a contentious view, perhaps, and one that cannot easily be demonstrated with our data. We suspect that, absent partisanship, many of our American respondents might feel differently about health care policy. But partisanship exists, and it colors the relationship between health care policy and a host of other variables. We cannot simply subtract it out. But doing so would, we suspect, change the distribution of opinion significantly.

TOWARD CONVERGENCE?

We wish to make three final points at the end of this long journey devoted to the examination of Americans' and Canadians' opinions about their health care system.

First, it is notable that one—if not *the*—central concern in attitudes about health care policy in both the US and Canada is about access to services. Those issues of access are different from one country to the next, of course: in the US the main concern has to do with inequality of access, whereas in Canada the main concern has to do with equal but slow access. This may be the central trade-off between private and public systems—the former tend to provide very good health care to a select few, while the latter provide care to everyone, but often have to limit quality in order to achieve this. (That this trade-off is so readily evident in our opinion data is testament, again, to the rationality of public opinion in salient policy domains.) But the idea that both systems are grappling with a similar issue, or, moreover, that *citizens* in both systems are grappling with a similar issue, is, we believe, both illuminating and instructive.

There are some important differences between American and Canadian attitudes toward health care, however. We have already noted several of these. But our second final point here is on another difference, most evident in Chapter 5; namely, the more structured character of Americans' opinions on health care. This structure comes, we believe, from a combination of partisanship/polarization and issue salience. Issue salience leads to more informed public opinion, and the current debate over health care reform in the US has certainly led to (somewhat) more informed attitudes. But the structure of Americans' attitudes toward health care is equally driven by the partisan nature of the debate. Our evidence makes clear that partisanship can have a powerful influence on policy attitudes. Whether that influence is positive (helpfully guiding) or negative (distracting) is another matter, of course. And one fact is clear: overall, Americans are less satisfied with their health care system than Canadians are, and they are more inclined to want a large-scale reform.

Our third and final point concerns the potential impact of mass opinion on the evolution of the health care system in the US and Canada. Our working hypothesis on that account is twofold. First, we suspect that in the future politicians, private interests, and governments will continue to exert a strong influence on citizens' opinions. There was, for instance, considerable strategic communication efforts invested by the Canadian government between 2005 and 2009 to improve public awareness of, and satisfaction with, Health Canada. The main objective was to "brand" Health Canada as "the steward and guardian of Canada's health care system and of the principles of Medicare" (Strategic Counsel 2009, 5). The US government has not yet invested comparable resources with the explicit objective of increasing Americans' satisfaction and loyalty with their health care system. But the role of partisanship makes clear the potential importance of elites in American health care policy. In the end, we believe elites' consensual politics in Canada and elites' polarized politics in the US will continue to structure both public policy and public opinion.

But we also think that the "autonomous" signal that comes from public opinion in the US and in Canada can eventually bring changes on both sides of the border. The outcome will likely be a greater convergence between both health care systems. The American system will move toward state-sponsored policies; Canada will flirt with privatization. Given the state of opinion in the US, convergence will be driven more by change in the American health care system than by change in Canada. This trend is already well underway, and the fact that these shifts can be predicted—or, at least, postdicted—by public attitudes about health care is no small matter. Clearly, public opinion and policy can be fundamentally intertwined. And public opinion—particularly well-informed opinion—often matters.

Appendix

Dependent Variables		
Satisfaction (CAN)	5-point scale	0 = very dissatisfied; 1 = very satisfied
Satisfaction (USA)	5-point scale	0 = very dissatisfied; 1 = very satisfied
OpinionUSA(CAN)	4-point scale	0 = very negative; 1 = very positive
OpinionUSA(CAN) (DK)	Dummy variable	1 = don't know; 0 = otherwise
OpinionCAN (USA)	4-point scale	0 = very negative; 1 = very positive
OpinionCAN(USA) (DK)	Dummy variable	1 = don't know; 0 = otherwise
Reforms (CAN)	3-point scale	0 = everything is fine or minor tune ups; 0.5 = fairly major repairs; 1 = complete rebuilding
Reforms (USA)	3-point scale	0 = everything is fine or minor tune ups; 0.5 = fairly major repairs; 1 = complete rebuilding
Socioeconomic Status Variables		
AB	Dummy variable	1 = resident of Alberta
BC	Dummy variable	1 = resident of British Columbia
QC	Dummy variable	1 = resident of Quebec
Prairies	Dummy variable	1 = resident of Manitoba or Saskatchewan
Atlantic	Dummy variable	1 = resident of Newfoundland or Prince Edward Island or Nova Scotia or New Brunswick
South	Dummy variable	1 = resident of one of the Southern U.S. states
Male	Dummy variable	1 = male
Age		Actual age of the respondent in 2011

Socioeconomic Status Variables		
Black	Dummy variable	1 = African American (U.S. only)
Education		Highest level of education completed 1 = less than elementary 2 = elementary school completed 3 = less than high school 4 = high school completed 5 = less than college/technical school/pre-university completed 6 = college/technical school/pre-university completed 7 = less than university completed 8 = university completed
Gvt. emp.	Dummy variable	1 = employed by the government
Income		Last year's total household income before taxes, which includes income from savings, pensions, rent, and wages. 1 = less than $20,000 2 = between $20,000 and $30,000 ($29,999) 3 = between $30,000 and $40,000 4 = between $40,000 and $50,000 5 = between $50,000 and $60,000 6 = between $60,000 and $70,000 7 = between $70,000 and $80,000 8 = between $80,000 and $90,000 9 = between $90,000 and $100,000 10 = between $100,000 and $110,000 11 = between $110,000 and $120,000 12 = more than $120,000
Medicare		1 = people in the U.S. who are covered by either Medicare or Medicaid
Personal Experience		
SatINS (US only)	3-point scale	Overall, are you very satisfied, fairly satisfied, fairly dissatisfied, or very dissatisfied with your current health insurance plan? 0 = fairly dissatisfied, very dissatisfied, DK 0.5 = fairly satisfied 1 = very satisfied

Personal Experience		
Past2years: egotropic (high)	5-point scale	Overall, how do you rate the quality of medical care that you and your family have received in the past 2 years from your doctor/GP/the place you usually go to? 0 = very poor 1 = excellent
Risk scale (high)		Comprised of series of "risk" variables asking about the risks that in the coming years a respondent or a family member will be unable to afford needed health care, get the most effective drugs, receive high-quality medical care, or wait longer than reasonable to get health care services. 0 = risk very low 1 = risk very high
Attitudes and Perceptions		
CANnopid	Dummy variable	1 = does not identify with a political party (Canada)
USAnopid	Dummy variable	1 = does not identify with a political party (USA)
Liberal	Dummy variable	1 = identifies with the Liberal Party
NDP	Dummy variable	1 = identifies with the NDP
Bloc	Dummy variable	1 = identifies with BQ
Green	Dummy variable	1 = identifies with the Green Party
Democrat	Dummy variable	1 = identifies with the Democratic Party
Ideology (right)	6-point scale	Self placement on the ideological scale 0 = left 1 = right
Ideology (conservative)	6-point scale	Self placement on the ideological scale 0 = liberal 1 = conservative
Government role (more)	5-point scale	0 = government lets each person get ahead on their own 1 = government sees that every person has a job and a good standard of living
Individualism scale (more)		0 = little individualistic 1 = very individualistic

Attitudes and Perceptions		
Gov. insurance plan	5-point scale	Some people say that there should be a government insurance plan, which would cover all medical and hospital expenses for everyone. Other people say that all medical expenses should be paid by individuals, and through private insurance plans like Blue Cross and other company-paid plans. And, of course, other people have opinions somewhere in between. Where would you place yourself on this scale, or haven't you thought much about this? 0 = all expenses paid by individuals and through private plans 1 = government insurance plan that covers all expenses for everyone
Universal access	5-point scale	Some people say that ensuring that health care is universally available to everyone, regardless of their ability to pay, is so important that we must do everything we can to protect these principles. Other people say that ensuring universal access, regardless of ability to pay, is simply too costly and we cannot afford to expect so much from the health care system. And, of course, other people have opinions somewhere in between. Where would you place yourself on this scale, or haven't you thought much about this? 0 = universal access is too costly and cannot be afforded 1 = do everything to protect principles of universal access
Public system: symbol		Universal publicly-funded health care is part of what it means to be Canadian and reflects our core values. 1 = people agreeing with the statement
Private system: symbol		Market-based health care is part of what it means to be American and reflects our core values. 1 = people agreeing with the statement
Health care system: symbol		Do you consider the health care system as a unifying symbol of your country and its people? 1 = yes

Attitudes and Perceptions	
Past2years: sociotropic (high) (Opinion about quality of HC in the past 2 years)	In your opinion, has the quality of health care in your country over the past two years deteriorated, improved or stayed the same? Please respond using a 5-point scale where 1 means greatly deteriorated, 5 greatly improved and 3 means stayed the same. 0 = 1,2 = greatly deteriorated 0.5 = 3 = remains the same 1 = 4,5 = greatly improved
Proplower (CAN)	Comprised of series of "proportion" questions, including whether the proportion of the population that had to wait longer than reasonable to get health care services in Canada is higher, lower, or about the same as in the United States. Other questions involve health care coverage, health care affordability, drugs, and access to high-quality medical care. (DK responses included with "same" responses.) 0 = proportion higher in Canada . . . 1 = proportion lower in Canada
Proplower (USA)	Comprised of series of "proportion" questions, including whether the proportion of the population that had to wait longer than reasonable to get health care services in Canada is higher, lower, or about the same as in the United States. Other questions involve health care coverage, health care affordability, drugs, and access to high-quality medical care. (DK responses included with "same" responses.) 0 = proportion higher in Canada . . . 1 = proportion lower in Canada

Attitudes and Perceptions	
BestsystemIND (CAN)	Comprised of series of "which system" variables pertaining to the respondent and his/her family, asking which health care system is better at dealing with issues of affordability, drugs, access to high-quality medical care, quick access to trained specialist, surgery as soon as possible, choice of hospital or doctor. (DK responses included as 0.5.) 0 = American system better . . . 1 = Canadian system better
BestsystemIND (USA)	Comprised of series of "which system" variables pertaining to the respondent and his/her family, asking which health care system is better at dealing with issues of affordability, drugs, access to high-quality medical care, quick access to trained specialist, surgery as soon as possible, choice of hospital or doctor. (DK responses included as 0.5.) 0 = American system better . . . 1 = Canadian system better
BestsystemPOP (CAN)	Comprised of series of "which system" variables pertaining to the population as a whole, asking which health care system is better at dealing with issues of affordability, drugs, access to high-quality medical care, quick access to trained specialist, surgery as soon as possible, choice of hospital or doctor. (DK responses included as 0.5.) 0 = American system better . . . 1 = Canadian system better

Attitudes and Perceptions		
BestsystemPOP (USA)		Comprised of series of "which system" variables pertaining to the population as a whole, asking which health care system is better at dealing with issues of affordability, drugs, access to high-quality medical care, quick access to trained specialist, surgery as soon as possible, choice of hospital or doctor. (DK responses included as 0.5.) 0 = American system better . . . 1 = Canadian system better
Opinion about own HCS (CAN)	5-point scale	0 = very dissatisfied; 1 = very satisfied
Opinion about own HCS (USA)	5-point scale	0 = very dissatisfied; 1 = very satisfied
Opinion about neighbor HCS (CAN)	5-point scale	0 = very dissatisfied; 1 = very satisfied
Opinion about HCS (USA)	5-point scale	0 = very dissatisfied; 1 = very satisfied

Bibliography

Adams, Michael. 2003. *Fire and Ice: The United States, Canada and the Myth of Converging Values*. Toronto: Penguin Canada.

Aldrich, John H., and James S. Coleman Battista. 2002. "Conditional Party Government in the States."*American Journal of Political Science* 46: 164–172.

Angus Reid. 2009. "Canadians, Americans Envy Different Aspects of the Health Care System." Angus Reid Report, August 6.

Baldassari, Delia, and Andrew Gelman. 2008. "Partisan without Constraint: Political Polarization and Trends in American Public Opinion." *American Journal of Sociology* 114: 408–446.

Bartels, Larry M. 2008. *Unequal Democracy: The Political Economy of the New Gilded Age*. Princeton: Princeton University Press.

Bélanger, Éric, and Richard Nadeau. 2009. *Le comportement électoral des Québécois*. Montréal: Presses de l'Université de Montréal.

Bélanger, Éric, and François Pétry. 2005. "The Rational Public? A Canadian Test of the Page and Shapiro Argument." *International Journal of Public Opinion Research* 17: 190–212.

Blais, André, Elisabeth Gidengil, Richard Nadeau, and Neil Nevitte. 2002. *Anatomy of a Liberal Victory: Making Sense of the Vote in the 2000 Canadian Election*. Peterborough: Broadview Press.

Blendon, Robert J., Drew E. Altman, John M. Benson, Mollyann Brodie, Tami Buhr, Claudia Deane, and Sasha Buscho. 2008. "Voters and Health Reform in the 2008 Presidential Election." *New England Journal of Medicine* 359: 2050–2061.

Blendon, Robert J., Drew E. Altman, Claudia Deane, John M. Benson, Mollyann Brodie, and Tami Buhr. 2008. "Health Care in the 2008 Presidential Primaries." *New England Journal of Medicine* 358: 414–422.

Blendon, Robert J., Robert Leitman, Ian Morrison, and Karen Donelan. 1990. "Satisfaction with Health Systems in Ten Nations." *Health Affairs* 9: 185–192.

Blendon, Robert J., Cathy Schoen, Catherine M. DesRoches, Robin Osborn, Kimberly L. Scoles, and Kinga Zapert. 2002. "Inequities in Health Care: A Five Country Study." *Health Affairs* 21: 182–191.

Blendon, Robert J., and Humphrey Taylor. 1989. "Views on Health Care: Public Opinion in Three Nations." *Health Affairs* 8: 149–157.

Blidook, Kelly. 2008. "Media, Public Opinion and Health Care in Canada: How the Media Affect 'The Way Things Are.' " *Canadian Journal of Political Science* 41: 355–374.

Bodenheimer, Thomas S., and Kevin Grumbach, K. 2012. *Understanding Health Policy: A Clinical Approach*, 6th ed. New York: Lange Medical Books McGraw-Hill.

Bothwell, Robert, and John English. 1981. "Pragmatic Physicians: Canadian Medicare and Health Care Insurance, 1910–1945." In S. E. D. Shortt, ed., *Medicine in*

Canadian Society: Historical Perspectives. Montreal: McGill-Queen's University Press, 479–493.

Boychuk, Gerard. 1998. *Patchworks of Purpose: The Development of Provincial Social Assistance Regimes in Canada*. Montreal: McGill-Queen's University Press.

Boychuk, Gerard. 2008. *National Health Insurance in the United States and Canada: Race, Territory and the Roots of Difference*. Washington, DC: Georgetown University Press.

Breton, Pascale. 2014. "Une opinion négative des soins de santé." *La Presse*, January 21, p.A15.

Brewer, Mark D. 2005. "The Rise of Partisanship and the Expansion of Partisan Conflict within the American Electorate." *Political Research Quarterly* 58: 219–229.

Bryden, Kenneth. 1974. *Old Age Pensions and Policy-Making in Canada*. Montreal: McGill-Queen's University Press.

Campbell, Angus, Philip E. Converse, Warren E. Miller, and Donald E. Stokes. 1960. *The American Voter*. New York: John Wiley and Sons.

Castonguay, Claude. 2008. *En avoir pour notre argent*. Rapport du Groupe de travail sur le financement du système de santé. Québec: Gouvernement du Québec.

Castonguay, Claude. 2012. *Santé: l'heure des choix*. Montréal: Boréal.

Chong, Dennis, and James N. Druckman. 2007. "Framing Theory." *Annual Review of Political Science* 10: 103–126.

Clair, Michel. 2001. *Emerging Solutions–Report and Recommendations*. Quebec: Commission d'étude sur les services de santé et les services sociaux.

Cochrane, Christopher. 2010. "Left/Right Ideology and Canadian Politics." *Canadian Journal of Political Science* 43: 583–605.

Commonwealth Fund. 2013. *International Profiles of Health Care Systems*. Commonwealth Fund Publication No. 1717.

Commonwealth Fund. 2014. *The Commonwealth Fund 2013 Annual Report*. New York: The Commonwealth Fund.

Delli Carpini, Michael X., and Scott Keeter. 1996. *What Americans Know about Politics and Why It Matters*. New Haven: Yale University Press.

Derthick, Martha. 1979. *Policymaking for Social Security*. Washington, DC: The Brookings Institution.

Entman, Robert M. 2004. *Projections of Power: Framing News, Public Opinion, and U.S. Foreign Policy*. Chicago: Chicago of University Press.

Gelman, Andrew, Daniel Lee, and Yair Ghitza. 2010. "Public Opinion on Health Care Reform." *The Forum*. www.bepress.com/forum/vol8/iss1/art8.

Gibbins, Roger, and Neil Nevitte. 1985. "Canadian Political Ideology: A Comparative Analysis." *Canadian Journal of Political Science* 18: 577–598.

Gidengil, Elisabeth, André Blais, Neil Nevitte, and Richard Nadeau. 2004. *Citizens*. Vancouver: UBC Press.

Grabb, Edward, and James Curtis. 2005. *Regions Apart: The Four Societies of Canada and the United States*. Don Mills: Oxford University Press.

Granatstein, J. L. 1986. *Canada 1957–1967: The Years of Uncertainty and Innovation*. Toronto: McClelland & Stewart.

Grayson, Linda, and Michael Bliss, eds. 1971. *The Wretched of Canada: Letters to R. B. Bennett 1930–1935*. Toronto: University of Toronto Press.

Hacker, Jacob. 1998. "The Historical Logic of National Health Insurance: Structure and Development of British, Canadian, and US Medical Policy." *Studies in American Political Development* 12: 57–130.

Hébert, Chantal. 2012. "Quebec Among Best Friends of Health Care System." *Toronto Star*, August 13. www.thestar.com/news/canada/politics/article/1241450—hebert-quebec-among-best-friends-of-health-care-system.

Jacobs, Lawrence R. 1992. "Institutions and Culture: Health Policy and Public Opinion in the U.S. and Britain." *World Politics* 44: 179–209.

Jacobs, Lawrence R. 2008. "1994 All Over Again? Public Opinion and Health Care." *New England Journal of Medicine* 358: 1881–1883.

Jacobs, Lawrence R., and Timothy Callaghan. 2013. "Why States Expand Medicaid: Party, Resources, and History." *Journal of Health Politics, Policy and Law* 38: 1023–1050.

Jacobs, Lawrence R., and Robert Y. Shapiro. 2000. *Politicians Don't Pander.* Chicago: University of Chicago Press.

Jacobs, Lawrence R., and Theda Skocpol. 2012. *Health Care Reforms and American Politics,* 2nd ed. New York: Oxford University Press.

Jacoby, William G. 2009. "Ideology and Vote Choice in the 2004 Election." *Electoral Studies* 28: 584–594.

Kaiser Family Foundation. 2010. "Medicaid Coverage and Spending in Health Reform." Available at: http://kaiserfamilyfoundation.files.wordpress.com/2013/01/medicaid-coverage-and-spending-in-health-reform-national-and-state-by-state-results-for-adults-at-or-below-133-fpl.pdf

Lasser, Karen E., David U. Himmelstein, and Steffie Woolhandler. 2006. "Access to Care, Health Status, and Health Disparities in the United States and Canada: Results of a Cross-National Population-Based Survey." *American Journal of Public Health* 96: 1300–1307.

Lazar, Harvey. 2009. "A Cross-Provincial Comparison of Health Care Reform in Canada: Building Blocs and Some Preliminary Results." *Canadian Political Science Review* 3: 1–14.

Lewis-Beck, Michael S. 1995. "Data Analysis: An Introduction." Sage University Paper Series in Quantitative Applications in Social Sciences, no. 103.

Lewis-Beck, Michael S., William G. Jacoby, Helmut Norpoth, and Herbert F. Weisberg. 2008. *The American Voter Revisited.* Ann Arbor: University of Michigan Press.

Lewis-Beck, Michael S., and Mary Stegmaier. 2007. "Economic Models of Voting." In Russell J. Dalton and Hans-Dieter Klingemann, eds., *The Oxford Handbook of Political Behavior.* Oxford: Oxford University Press, 518–537.

Lipset, Seymour M. 1983. "Roosevelt and the Protest of the 1930s." *Minnesota Law Review* 68: 273–298.

Lipset, Seymour M. 1990. *Continental Divide: The Values and Institutions of the United States and Canada.* New York: Routledge.

Maioni, Antonia. 1998. *Parting at the Crossroads: The Emergence of Health Insurance in the United States and Canada.* Princeton, NJ: Princeton University Press.

Maioni, Antonia. 2009. "Health Care Reform in the 2008 US Presidential Election." *International Journal* 64: 135–144.

Maioni, Antonia, and Pierre Martin. 2004. "Public Opinion and Health Care Reform in Canada: Exploring the Sources of Discontent." Paper presented at the annual meeting of the American Political Science Association, Chicago (September 1–5).

Marmor, Theodore R. 1973. *The Politics of Medicare.* Chicago: Aldine.

Marmor, Theodore R. 1993. "Health Care Reform in the United States: Patterns of Facts and Fiction in the Use of Canadian Experience." *American Review of Canadian Studies* 23: 47–64.

Marmor, Theodore R., and Jonathan Oberlander. 2011. "The Patchwork: Health Reform, American Style." *Social Science & Medicine* 72: 125–128.

Mauser, Gary. 1990. "A Comparison of Canadian and American Attitudes Towards Firearms." *Canadian Journal of Criminology* 32: 573–589.

Mauser, Gary, and Michael Margolis. 1992. "The Politics of Gun Control: Comparing Canadian and American Patterns." *Government and Policy* 10: 189–209.

McCarty, Nolan, Keith Poole, and Howard Rosenthal. 2008. *Polarized America: The Dance of Ideology and Unequal Riches.* Cambridge, MA: MIT Press.

McClosky, Herbert, and John Zaller. 1984. *The American Ethos: Public Attitudes towards Capitalism and Democracy.* Cambridge: Cambridge University Press.

Mendelsohn, Matthew. 2002. "Canadians' Thoughts on Their Health Care System: Preserving the Canadian Model through Innovation." Report for the Commission on the Future of Health Care in Canada. Ottawa: Government of Canada.

Miller, Warren E., and J. Merrill Shanks. 1996. *The New American Voter.* Cambridge: Harvard University Press.

Morone, James A. 2010. "Presidents and Health Reform: From Franklin D. Roosevelt To Barack Obama." *Health Affairs* 29: 1096–1100.

Morone, James A., and Lawrence R. Jacobs, eds. 2005. *Healthy, Wealthy, and Fair: Health Care and the Good Society.* New York: Oxford University Press.

Nadeau, Richard, and Éric Bélanger. 2013. "Un modèle général d'explication du vote des Québécois." In Frédérick Bastien, Éric Bélanger, and François Gélineau, eds., *Les Québécois aux urnes.* Montreal: Presses de l'Université de Montréal, 191–207.

Nadeau, Richard, Éric Bélanger, and Bruno Jérôme (2012). "The Economy and Federal Election Outcomes in Canada: Taking Provincial Economic Conditions into Account." Paper presented at the conference on *Duty and Choice: Participation and Preferences in Democratic Elections*, Montreal, Canada.

Nadeau, Richard, Éric Bélanger, Michael S. Lewis-Beck, Bruno Cautrès, and Martial Foucault. 2012. *Le vote des Français de Mitterrand à Sarkozy.* Paris: Presses de Sciences Po.

Nadeau, Richard, and André Blais. 1995. "Economic Conditions, Leader Evaluations and Election Outcomes in Canada." *Canadian Public Policy* 21: 212–218.

Nadeau, Richard, Michael S. Lewis-Beck, and Éric Bélanger. 2013. "Economics and Elections Revisited." *Comparative Political Studies* 46: 551–573.

Nadeau, Richard, Neil Nevitte, Elisabeth Gidengil, and André Blais. 2008. "Election Campaigns as Information Campaigns: Who Learns What and Does It Matter?" *Political Communication* 25: 229–248.

Nadeau, Richard, François Pétry, and Éric Bélanger. 2010. "Strategic Issue Framing in Election Campaigns: The Case of Health Care in the 2000 Canadian Federal Election." *Political Communication* 27: 367–388.

Nesbitt-Larking, Paul. 2002. "Canadian Political Culture: The Problem of Americanization." In Mark Charlton and Paul Barker, eds., *Crosscurrents: Contemporary Political Issues,* 4th ed. Toronto: ITP Nelson, 4–21.

New York Times. 2009. "Obama, Armed With Details, Says Health Plan Is Necessary." September 9. www.nytimes.com/2009/09/10/us/politics/10obama.html?pagewanted=all&_r=0

Numbers, Ronald. 1978. *Almost Persuaded: American Physicians and Compulsory Health Insurance, 1912–1920.* Baltimore: Johns Hopkins University Press.

OECD. (2011). "Health at a Glance: 2011: OECD Indicators." OECD Publishing. http://dx.doi.org/10.1787/health_glance-2011-en.

Page, Benjamin I., and Robert Y. Shapiro. 1992. *The Rational Public.* Chicago: University of Chicago Press.

Perlin, George. 1997. "The Constraints of Public Opinion: Diverging or Converging Paths?" In Keith Banting, George Hoberg, and Richard Simeon, eds., *Degrees of Freedom: Canada and the United States in a Changing World.* Montreal: McGill-Queen's University Press, 71–149.

Pétry, François, and Matthew Mendelsohn. 2004. "Public Opinion and Policy Making in Canada." *Canadian Journal of Political Science* 37: 505–530.

Popkin, Samuel L. 1991. *The Reasoning Voter: Communication and Persuasion in Presidential Campaigns.* Chicago: University of Chicago Press.

Romanow, Roy J. 2002. *Building on Values: The Future of Health Care in Canada–Final Report.* Ottawa: Commission on the Future of Health Care in Canada.

Sanmartin, Claudia, Jean-Marie Berhtolot, Edward Ng, Kellie Murphy, Debra L. Blackwell, Jane F. Gentleman, Michael E. Martinez, and Catherine M. Simile. 2006. "Comparing Health and Health Care Use in Canada and the United States." *Health Affairs* 25: 1133–1140.

Savoie, Donald J. 1999. *Governing from the Centre: The Concentration of Power in Canadian Politics*. Toronto: University of Toronto Press.

Schiltz, Michael. 1970. *Public Attitudes Toward Social Security, 1935–1965*. Washington: U.S. Department of Health, Education, and Welfare, Social Security Administration, Office of Research and Statistics (Research Report No. 33).

Schlesinger, Mark, and Richard R. Lau. 2000. "The Meaning and Measure of Policy Metaphors." *American Political Science Review* 94: 611–626.

Schlesinger, Mark, and Teaku Lee. 1993. "Is Health Care Different? Popular Support of Federal Health and Social Policies." *Journal of Health Politics, Policy and Law* 18: 551–628.

Simpson, Jeffrey. 2000. *Star-Spangled Canadians*. Toronto: HarperCollins.

Sniderman, Paul M., Richard A. Brody, and Philip E. Tetlock. 1991. *Reasoning and Choice: Explorations in Political Psychology*. New York: Cambridge University Press.

Soroka, Stuart. 2002. *Agenda-Setting Dynamics in Canada*. Vancouver: University of British Columbia Press.

Soroka, Stuart. 2007. *Canadian Perceptions of the Health Care System: A Report to the Health Council of Canada*. Toronto: Health Council of Canada.

Soroka, Stuart, and Patrick Fournier. 2011. *The Sources of Public Attitudes on the Canadian Health Care System: A Report to the Canada Health Services Research Foundation*. Toronto: CHSRF.

Soroka, Stuart, and Elvin Lim. 2003. "Issue Definition and the Opinion-Policy Link: Public Preferences and Health Care Spending in the US and the UK." *British Journal of Politics and International Relations* 5: 576–593.

Soroka, Stuart, Antonia Maioni, and Pierre Martin. 2013. "What Moves Public Opinion on Health Care? Individual Experiences, System Performance, and Media Framing." *Journal of Health Politics, Policy and Law* 38: 893–920.

Soroka, Stuart, and Christopher Wlezien. 2010. *Degrees of Democracy: Politics, Public Opinion, and Policy*. New York: Cambridge University Press.

Starr, Paul. 1982. *The Social Transformation of American Medicine*. New York: Basic Books.

Strategic Counsel. 2009. *Health Canada Performance Survey 2009* (HC POR 08–18).

Stokes, Donald E. (1963). "Spatial Models of Party Competition." *American Political Science Review* 57: 368–377.

Sundquist, James L. 1968. *Politics and Policy: The Eisenhower, Kennedy and Johnson Years*. Washington, DC: The Brookings Institution.

Tuohy, Caroline. 1999. *Accidental Logics: The Dynamics of Change in the Health Care Arena in the United States, Britain and Canada*. New York: Oxford University Press.

Vavreck, Lynn. 2009. *The Message Matters: The Economy and Presidential Campaigns*. Princeton: University of Princeton Press.

Walker, Forrest A. 1969. "Compulsory Health Insurance: The Next Great Step in Social Legislation." *Journal of American History* 56: 290–304.

Wooldridge, Jeffrey M. 2006. *Introductory Econometrics: A Modern Approach*, 3rd ed. Mason, OH: Thomson/South-Western.

Zaller, John R. 1992. *The Nature and Origins of Mass Opinion*. Cambridge: Cambridge University Press.

Zaller, John R., and Stanley Feldman. 1992. "A Simple Theory of the Survey Response: Answering Questions versus Revealing Preferences." *American Journal of Political Science* 36: 579–616.

Zucker, Harold G. 1978. "The Variable Nature of News Influence." In B.D. Riben, ed., *Communications Yearbook,* vol 2. New Brunswick, NJ: Transaction Books, 225–245.

Index

For Product Safety Concerns and Information please contact our EU
representative GPSR@taylorandfrancis.com
Taylor & Francis Verlag GmbH, Kaufingerstraße 24, 80331 München, Germany

www.ingramcontent.com/pod-product-compliance
Ingram Content Group UK Ltd.
Pitfield, Milton Keynes, MK11 3LW, UK
UKHW021959180926
475701UK00003B/94

* 9 7 8 1 1 3 8 2 1 8 4 8 2 *